The Pocket Atlas of Special Tests for the Upper Limb

Jane Johnson

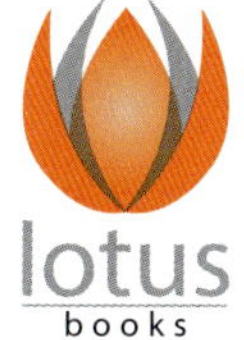

Library of Congress Cataloging-in-Publication Data

Names: Johnson, Jane, 1965- author.
Title: The pocket atlas of special tests for the upper limb / Jane Johnson.
Other titles: Special tests for the upper limb
Description: Champaign, Illinois : Lotus Books, 2026. | Includes bibliographical references.
Identifiers: LCCN 2025002854 (print) | LCCN 2025002855 (ebook) | ISBN 9781718243095 (paperback) | ISBN 9781718243101 (epub) | ISBN 9781718243118 (PDF)
Subjects: MESH: Musculoskeletal Diseases--diagnosis | Physical Examination--methods | Upper Extremity | Handbook
Classification: LCC RD557 (print) | LCC RD557 (ebook) | NLM WE 39 | DDC 617.5/7075--dc23/eng/20250402
LC record available at https://lccn.loc.gov/2025002854
LC ebook record available at https://lccn.loc.gov/2025002855

ISBN: 978-1-7182-4309-5 (print)

Illustrations (cover and interior) Amanda Williams and Lee Lawrence
Text Design Medlar Publishing Solutions Pvt Ltd., India
Cover Design Keri Evans
Printed By Versa Press

Printed in the United States of America 10 9 8 7 6 5 4 3 2 1

The paper in this book is certified under a sustainable forestry program.

Lotus Books
An Imprint of Human Kinetics
1607 N. Market Street
Champaign, IL 61820
USA

United States and International
Website: **US.HumanKinetics.com/pages/lotus-books**
Email: info@hkusa.com
Phone: 1-800-747-4457

Canada
Website: **Canada.HumanKinetics.com**
Email: info@hkcanada.com

Human Kinetics' authorized representative for product safety in the EU is Mare Nostrum Group B.V., Mauritskade 21D, 1091 GC Amsterdam, The Netherlands.
Email: gpsr@mare-nostrum.co.uk

L1178

Contents

Arrow Color Code

Green = Force/direction of movement by the client

Blue = Force/direction of movement by the clinician

Introduction

The Pocket Atlas of Special Tests for the Upper Limb is designed for use by manual therapists—physiotherapists, osteopaths, chiropractors, sports therapists—and by anyone who needs to assess someone with a musculoskeletal problem.

There is no agreed definition of what constitutes a "special" test in musculoskeletal assessment. These types of tests tend to be those that help us to identify with which structure a problem lies, and the name of the test has often been attributed to the person who first described it.

The text covers tests for the shoulder (Part I), the elbow (Part II), and the wrist and hand (Part III) and it is hoped that by using this book, you will find at least one of the 83 tests helpful in deciding whether a problem is likely to be with a joint, a ligament, a muscle or its tendon. Whilst most tests included here focus specifically on an assessment of the musculoskeletal system, seven tests have been included as being likely to be of help in assessing nerve compression at the elbow and wrist.

This book is intended as a quick reference guide, something you can use to familiarize yourself with the tests and how they are performed. It is not intended to be prescriptive as to which tests you should or should not use. Not all special tests have been rigorously assessed for validity and reliability. This book includes a wide range of tests, even those for which sensitivity or specificity has been found to be low. The reason for this is that you will almost certainly come across these tests at some point in your career, and it is important to make up your own mind as to the value of each, whilst taking into account the evidence from current research. You may even decide it is worth conducting research yourself into a particular test. Wherever possible, a reference has been cited relating to a test so that you can use this as a starting point for further research.

It is unlikely that any single test would be adequate to determine which shoulder, elbow, wrist, or hand structures are affected, which is why the use of multiple different tests is needed. It is likely that, due to time constraints, you will select those tests most likely to be appropriate, following the initial history you have taken from your client.

One of the problems identified with some of the tests described here is that they may have been modified (either in the literature or anecdotally) from what was originally described by the person to whom the test is attributed. Wherever possible, the description of the test is based on the description provided by the person to whom the test is attributed.

Another problem is that the original description may not have been precise. The Yergason Test for the shoulder is a good example. Yergason's Test is based on a single case study and the original paper describes the test but contains no illustration. In this example, the position intended for the therapists' hands is unknown. Clinician's regularly propose new assessments and it may be that when trying out some of the tests described here, you too come up with a novel approach that furthers the practice of manual assessment.

PART I

THE SHOULDER

The shoulder "complex" comprises the bones of the clavicle, scapula, humerus, and manubrium and the joints they form (figure I.1). Three of these joints are synovial—the acromioclavicular (AC) joint, the glenohumeral joint, and the sternoclavicular joint. The shoulder complex also includes the scapulothoracic joint, which is a functional joint formed by the motion of the scapula as it slides over the thorax.

Together these joints permit a wide range of movement for the upper limb but at the expense of stability.

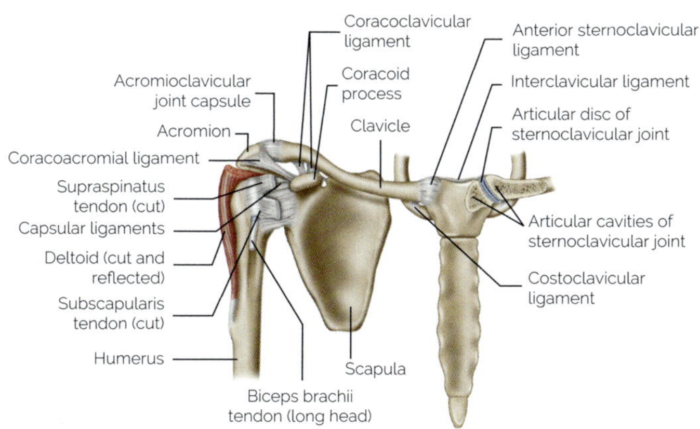

Figure I.1: The shoulder complex.

Shoulder stability is provided by muscles acting on the joints, rather than by the structure of the joints themselves (figure I.2).

In this part of the book, you will find 49 special tests to help you to test the joints and muscles of the shoulder complex. Tests include those used to assess the AC joint (chapter 1), the scapulothoracic joint (chapter 2), muscles of the rotator cuff (chapters 3, 4 and 5), the glenohumeral labrum and the long head of biceps brachii (chapter 6), plus a series of tests specific for assessing shoulder instability (chapter 7).

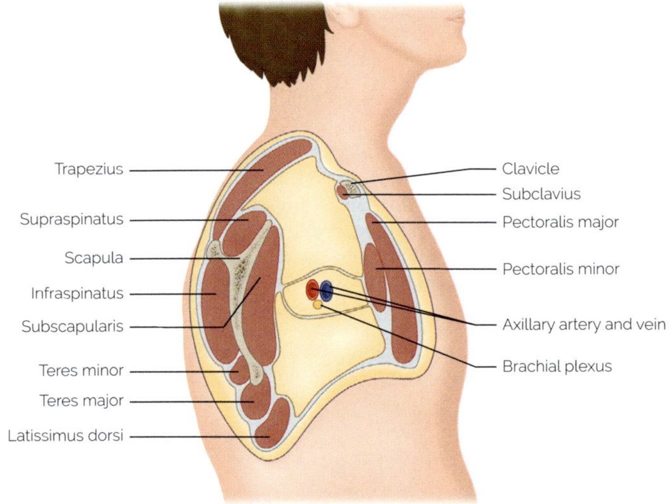

Figure I.2: Muscles of the shoulder.

CHAPTER 1

Acromioclavicular Joint

The small AC joint is formed by the attachment of the distal end of the clavicle with the acromion process of the scapula (figure 1.1). Every time we move our shoulders, the AC joint moves. You can test this for yourself by grasping your right clavicle between the thumb and forefinger of your left hand. Next, elevate and depress your right shoulder, protract and retract the shoulder, and notice that the clavicle moves all the time that you are moving your shoulder.

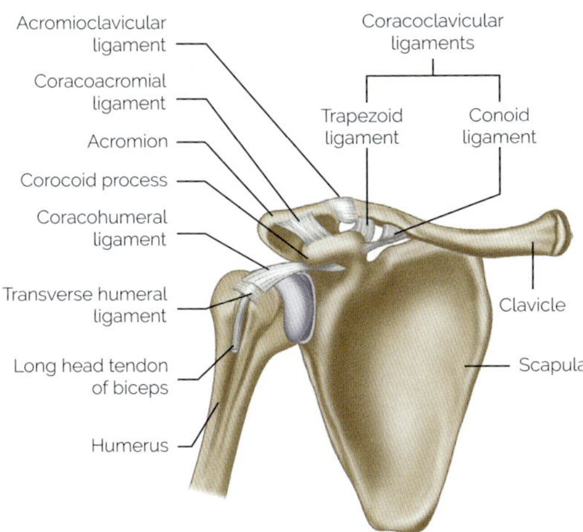

Figure 1.1: The AC joint and associated ligaments.

The need to facilitate movement leaves the AC joint vulnerable to injury. The coracoclavicular ligament is an important ligament providing stability for the joint by fixing the clavicle to the coracoid process of the scapula. It is made up of the trapezoid and conoid ligaments. The superior and inferior AC ligaments fix the clavicle to the acromion of the scapula. The AC joint is a plane synovial joint and may contain an articular disc.

Injuries to the AC ligaments are common. This chapter begins with a table setting out the grading used to describe AC joint ligament injuries, followed by seven special tests. These are the AC Mobility Test, the AC Shear Test, Paxino's Test, the Scarf Test (which you may know as the Cross-Body Adduction Stress Test), O'Brien's Test (also known as the Active Compression Test), the Resisted AC Joint Extension Test, and finally the Painful Arc Test.

Note that there are two painful arc tests included in this book, one for the AC joint as described in this chapter, and one for supraspinatus (described in chapter 3).

Grades of AC Joint Ligament Injury

Sprains of the AC joint are classified according to the severity of injury to the ligaments and joint capsule (table 1.1). Tossy, Mead, and Sigmond (1963) and Allman (1967) devised three grades of AC joint injury. Rockwood expanded on these and added a further three grades. These classifications were based on radiographic findings; clinical findings vary. For example, the specific site and severity of pain vary.

A useful overview of the Rockwood Classification of AC Joint Separations is provided by Gorbaty, Hsu, and Gee (2017).

In addition to the tests provided in this section, when working with sporting populations consider using a functional outcome score such as the Nottingham Clavicle Score (Charles et al. 2017).

Table 1.1: Classification of AC injuries.

Classification	Degree of Injury	Joint Laxity
Grade I	Only a few fibers of the AC ligament and capsule are torn	None
Grade II	Complete tear of the AC ligament; sprain of the coracoclavicular ligaments	Laxity frequently causing deformity, with the acromion sitting slightly higher than the clavicle; may be referred to as *minor subluxation*
Grade III	Rupture of both the AC and coracoclavicular ligaments	Obvious deformity: the distal end of the clavicle is palpable; may be referred to as dislocation; distal end of the clavicle is displaced superiorly
Grade IV	Rupture of both the AC and coracoclavicular ligaments	Dislocation of the AC joint with the end of the clavicle displaced posteriorly into the trapezius muscle
Grade V	Rupture of both the AC and coracoclavicular ligaments	Dislocation of the AC joint with the lateral end of the clavicle obviously displaced; possible disruption of deltoid and trapezial fascia
Grade VI	Rupture of both the AC and coracoclavicular ligaments	Dislocation of the AC joint with the lateral end of the clavicle displaced inferior to the acromion process; likely disruption of deltoid and trapezial fascia

AC Joint Mobility Test

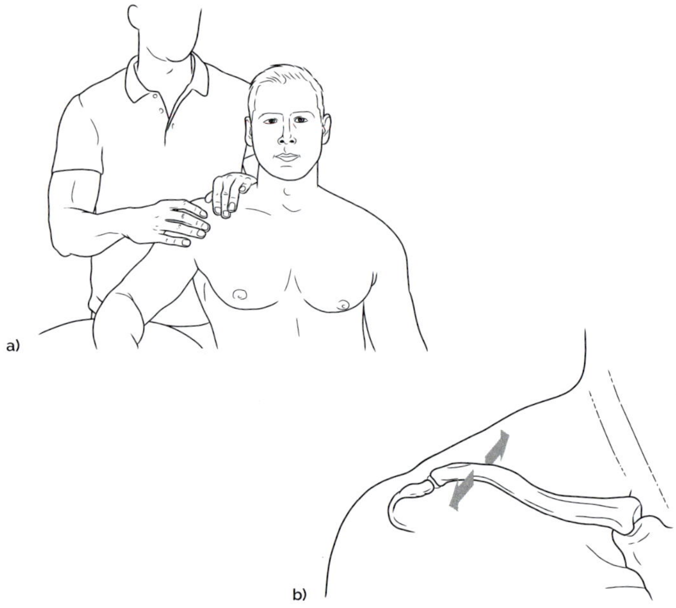

Figure 1.2: The AC Joint Mobility Test: (a) hand position; (b) movement of the clavicle against the acromion.

Purpose: This tests for laxity in the AC joint.

Type of Test: This is a passive test of AC joint mobility as well as a pain-provocation test.

Procedure: With your client seated, passively abduct the arm to about 20° by resting it on a plinth (figure 1.2a). Locate the AC joint. With one hand hold the acromion, and with the other pinch the distal end of the clavicle between your finger and thumb. Attempt to move the clavicle against the acromion, ventrally and dorsally (figure 1.2b).

Findings: There are a range of possible findings. No movement suggests the joint is intact. By contrast, where there is AC and coracoclavicular separation, the clavicle is displaced superiorly owing to the pull of the neck muscles. In this case, the clavicle can be pressed inferiorly.

Tip: This is easier to perform than Paxino's Test, which requires the examiner to use only one hand.

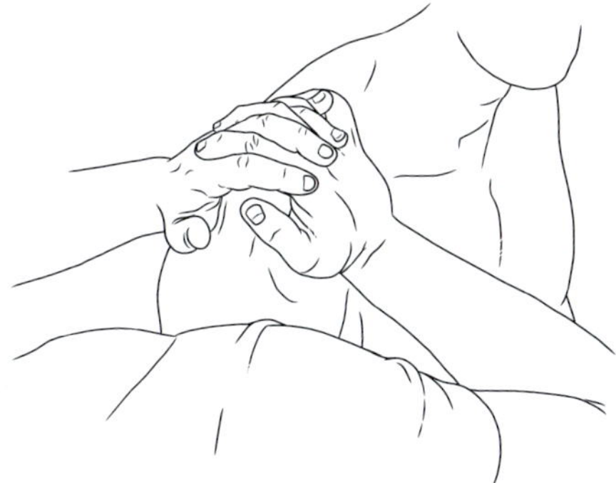

Figure 1.3: AC Shear Test.

Purpose: This tests for AC joint pathology.

Type of Test: This is a passive test of AC joint mobility as well as a pain-provocation test.

Procedure: Stand side-on to your client as they sit on a chair or the edge of a treatment plinth. Cup your hands around the shoulder, one hand on the spine of the scapula and one on the clavicle (figure 1.3). Gently squeeze the heels of your hands together.

Findings: The test is positive if there is pain localized to the AC joint.

Paxino's Test

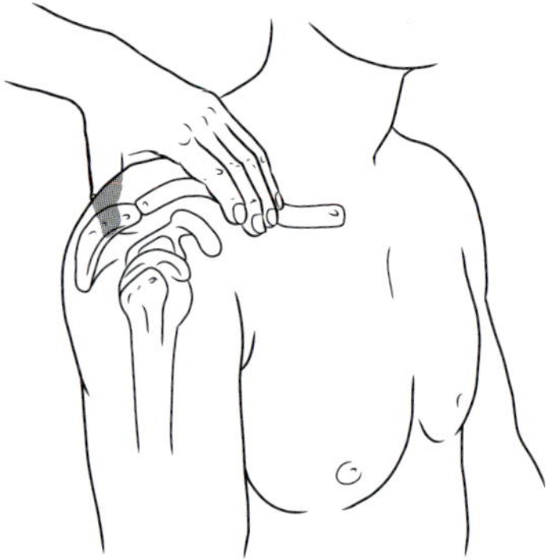

Figure 1.4: Paxino's Test.

Purpose: Described by Walton et al. (2004), this tests for pathology affecting the AC joint.

Type of Test: This is a passive pain-provocation test.

Procedure: With the client seated, place your thumb on the posterolateral aspect of the acromion on the affected shoulder, and one or more fingers superior to the midpart of the clavicle (figure 1.4).

Apply pressure with the thumb in an anterosuperior direction whilst simultaneously applying pressure inferiorly to the clavicle using your fingers.

Findings: The test is positive if it elicits pain in the AC joint.

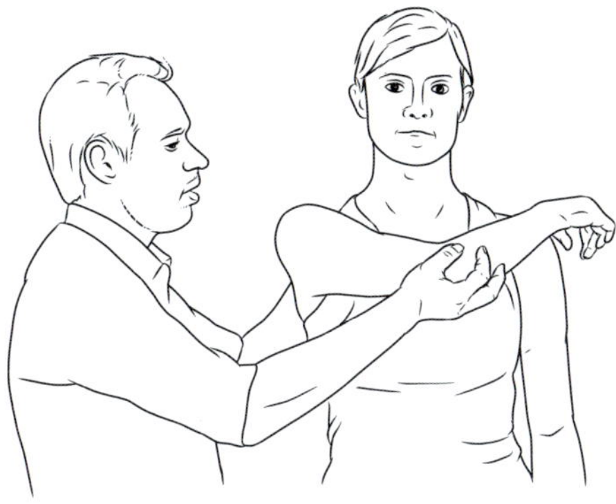

Figure 1.5: Scarf Test.

Purpose: This tests for integrity of the AC joint.

Type of Test: This is a passive pain-provocation test.

Procedure: Passively flex the client's arm to 90°. Stabilize the scapula using your other hand. Passively adduct the arm (figure 1.5), taking care to prevent rotation of the torso. This compresses the AC joint.

Findings: The test is positive if there is pain.

Tip: You may need to experiment with the position of the hand you use to support the elbow.

O'Brien's (Active Compression) Test

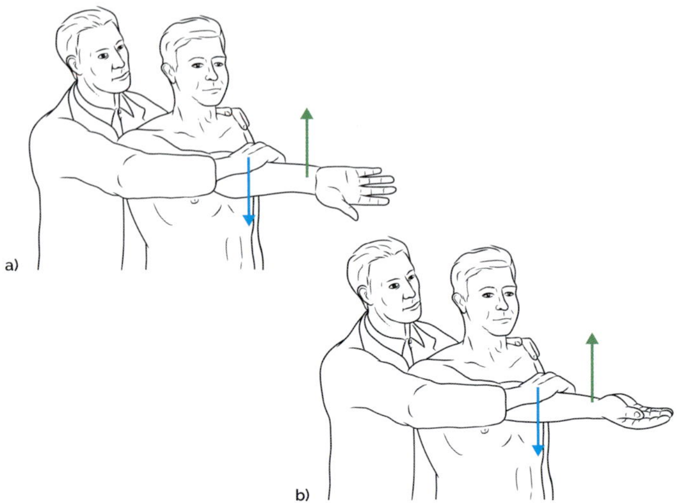

Figure 1.6: O'Brien's Test with the client's shoulder in full internal rotation (a) and full supination (b).

Purpose: Described by O'Brien et al. (1998), this tests for lesions of the AC joint and labrum of the glenohumeral joint.

Type of Test: This is a pain provocation test requiring muscle contraction against resistance.

Procedure: Ask your client to flex the shoulder to 90° and adduct it to 10°–15°.

From this starting point, there are then two test positions. First, ask your client to internally rotate their shoulder as fully as possible, pronating the forearm so that the thumb is pointing downward. Apply downward force to the distal forearm and ask your client to resist this (figure 1.6a). In this position, pressure increases in the AC joint.

Next, ask your client to fully supinate the forearm and to again resist the downward pressure that you apply (figure 1.6b).

Findings: The test is positive if pain elicited in the first maneuver is reduced or even eliminated in the second maneuver.
Pain localized to the AC joint indicates pathology. Pain or pain with clicking localized to the glenohumeral joint indicates a problem with the labrum.

Tip: Notice that placing one hand on the patient's nonaffected shoulder helps stabilize their torso.

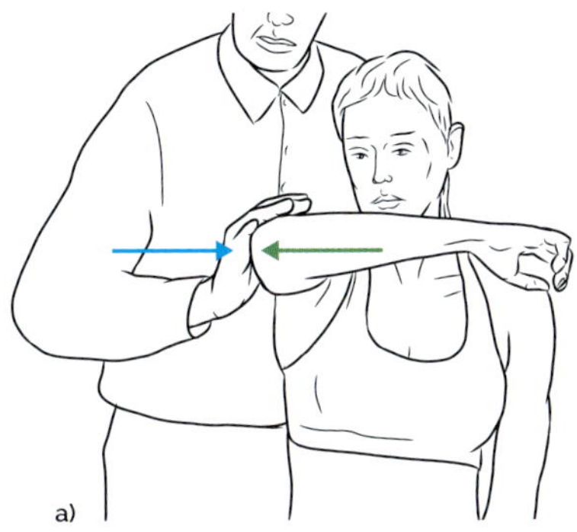

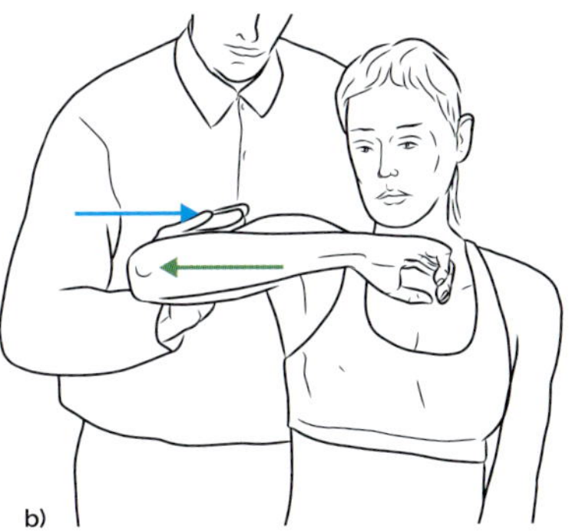

Figure 1.7: Resisted AC Joint Extension Test: (a) start position; (b) through greater degrees of horizontal extension.

Purpose: This tests for AC joint pathology.

Type of Test: This is a pain provocation test requiring muscle contraction against resistance.

Procedure: Begin with your client seated, with the shoulder flexed to 90° and internally rotated (figure 1.7a). Ask your client to horizontally abduct their am whilst you apply an isometric resistance.

Findings: The test is positive if there is pain at the AC joint.

Tip: Perform this test through a range of horizontal abduction. Note that in figure 1.7b the arm is more horizontally abducted than in figure 1.7a.

Painful Arc Test

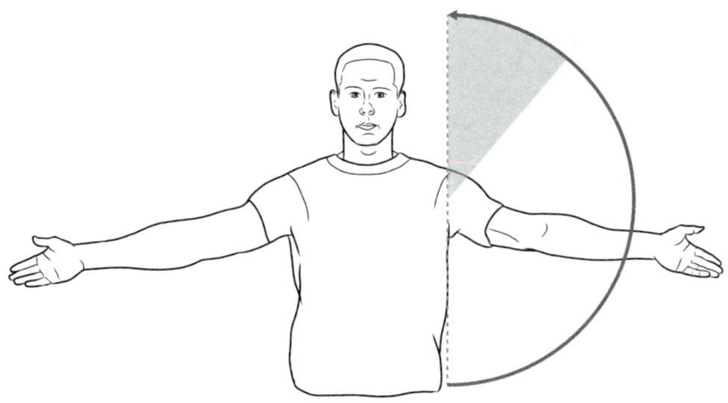

Figure 1.8: Painful Arc Test.

Purpose: This tests for AC joint pathology.

Type of Test: This is a pain provocation test requiring active muscle contraction, but which may also be performed passively.

Procedure: Ensure your client begins with a good, upright sitting or standing posture, as protraction of the scapula affects the test result. The client's arm is abducted either actively or passively through the full range of motion (ROM) (figure 1.8). The test is performed passively if the client does not have the muscle strength to move their arm through a full range.

Findings: At the upper end of elevation—between 140° and 180° of elevation—the acromion is compressed. The test is therefore positive for pathology of the AC joint if there is pain within this range.

Tip: This test is also used for impingement of the supraspinatus tendon, which elicits pain within the 70°–120° range. Other shoulder pathologies also give rise to a pain in shoulder abduction.

CHAPTER 2

Scapulothoracic Joint

The scapulothoracic joint is a functional joint formed by the sliding of the scapula over the thorax. It is classified as a "false" joint because it lacks a joint capsule, synovial membrane, synovial fluid, as well as ligamentous support.

Movement of this joint combined with movement of the glenohumeral joint is known as *scapulohumeral rhythm*. To fully elevate the arm, both the scapula and the glenohumeral joint must move. The scapula needs to move through 60°, whilst the glenohumeral joint simultaneously needs to move through 120° (figure 2.1). This requires mobility in both the AC and sternoclavicular joints.

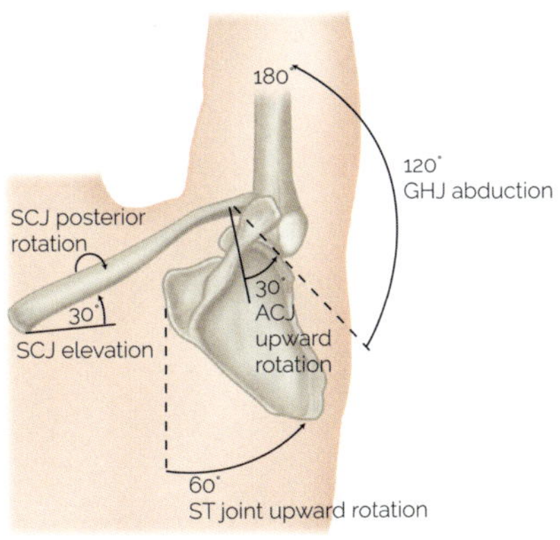

Figure 2.1: Scapulohumeral rhythm.

Whilst scapulohumeral rhythm varies between individuals, there are significant differences in movement of the scapula in people with a rotator cuff tear compared with those without.

Assessment of scapular movement may therefore be helpful as part of an overall shoulder assessment. In this chapter you will find three special tests commonly used to assess scapulothoracic movement. These are Apley's Scratch Test, the Lateral Scapular Slide Test, and the Scapular Assistance Test.

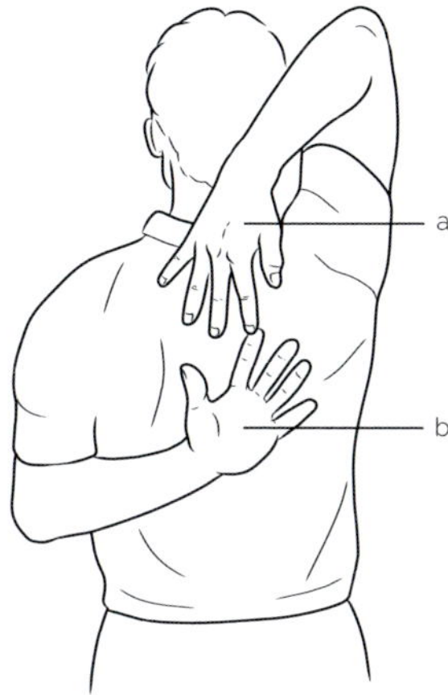

Figure 2.2: Apley's Scratch Test involves trying to reach over the head to touch the upper back with the palm of one hand (a) and reaching up the back with the dorsum of the other hand (b).

Purpose: Named after the British orthopedic surgeon Alan Graham Apley, this tests for range of movement in the shoulder.

Type of Test: This is a functional test of joint mobility, combining the glenohumeral, AC, and scapulothoracic joints.

Procedure: Ask your client to take one hand above their head, trying to reach the center of the upper back (figure 2.2a)—this tests lateral rotation with flexion and abduction. Then ask them to take the other hand behind their back, placing the dorsum of the hand against the back (figure 2.2b)—this tests medial rotation with extension and adduction.

The client should then reverse their hands and attempt the maneuver again, thus testing both shoulders for each combination of movements.

Findings: This is a quick functional test that can be made more objective by measuring either the distance between the fingertips or, for the lower hand, the distance between the fingertip and vertebra C7.

Lateral Scapular Slide Test

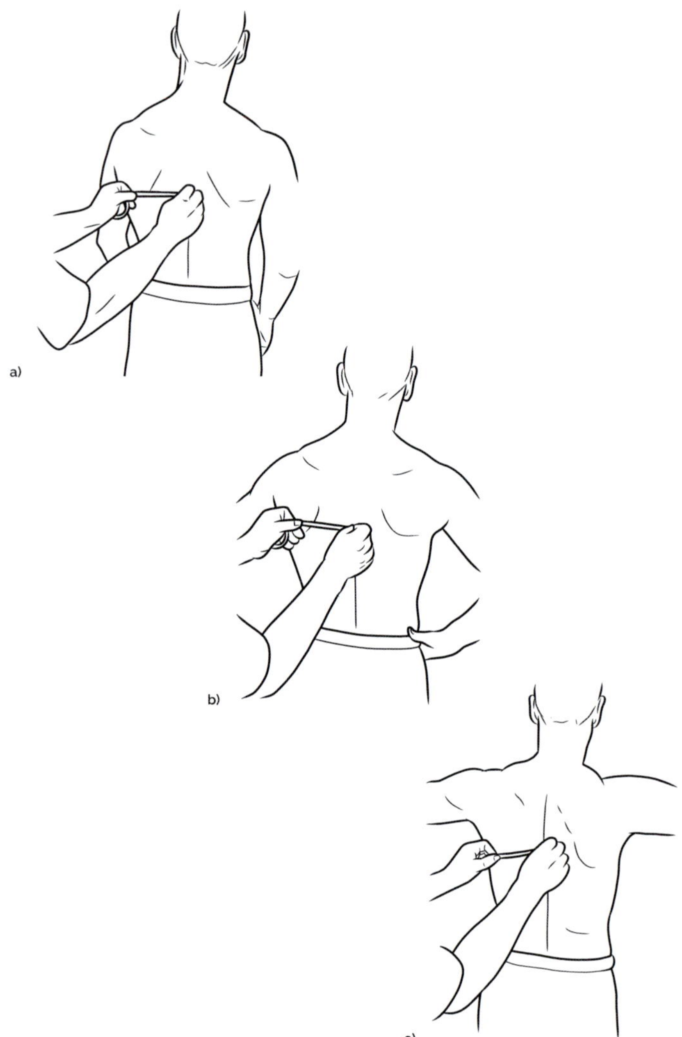

Figure 2.3: Lateral Scapular Slide Test: (a) start position with hands by the sides; (b) with hands on hips; (c) with the arms abducted.

Purpose: Described by Kibler (1998), this tests for stability of the scapula during movements of the glenohumeral joint.

Type of Test: This is a functional test of scapular stability requiring both concentric and eccentric muscle contraction.

Procedure: Varying arm positions progressively increase the load on the muscles of scapular stabilization, and for this reason it is important to perform the test in all three positions. Kibler advises that the test should be performed in both the ascending and descending phase of the arm in abduction and adduction, and when flexing and lowering the arm.

In the start position, your client stands with their hands resting by their sides; mark and measure the inferomedial angle of each scapula with respect to the closest spinous process (figure 2.3a). Mark also the spinous process.

In the second position the hands rest on the hips, thumbs posterior and fingers anterior, with the shoulder in about 10° of extension. Palpate the inferomedial aspect of the scapula, and measure this with respect to the original spinous process (figure 2.3b). In the third position, the arms are held at or below 90°, maximally internally rotated so that the thumbs are pointing downward, and the distance from the inferomedial aspect of the scapula is again measured (figure 2.3c). In each of the three positions check for asymmetry between left and right scapulae.

Findings: Weakness is indicated by asymmetry in the distance between the inferomedial angle of the left and right scapulae and the marked spinous process in each of the test positions.

In the start position (figure 2.3a) minimal muscle action is required. In the second position (figure 2.3b) the lower fibers of trapezius and serratus anterior are working at a low level to stabilize the scapula. Therefore, asymmetry in this position relates to those muscles. In the third position (figure 2.3c) upper trapezius, lower trapezius, serratus anterior, and rhomboids are working at about 40 percent of their maximum.

Tip: Weakness in scapular stabilizers is often noted as the arms are lowered.

Scapular Assistance Test

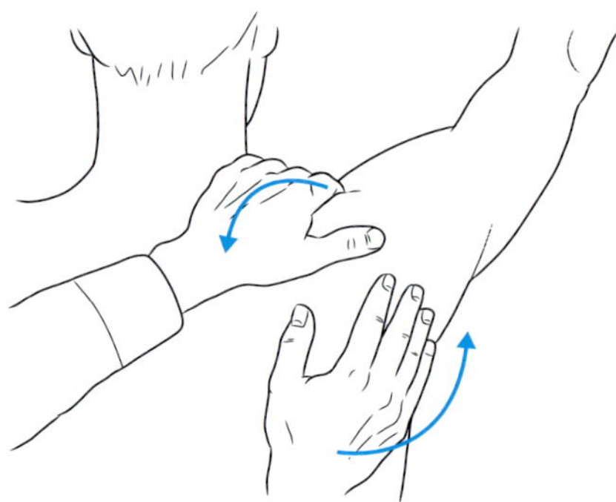

Figure 2.4: Scapular Assistance Test.

Purpose: Described by Kibler (1998), this test helps determine whether impingement at the shoulder may be due to a lack of active acromial elevation.

Type of Test: This is a muscle assistance test.

Procedure: This test is designed to work by mimicking the action of the muscles that would normally bring about scapular movement, as when the arm is raised. Rabin et al. (2006) described a modified version in which the tipping motion of the scapula was also simulated.

Your client stands with their hands by their sides. Place one of your hands over the superior angle of the scapula and the other hand such that the heel of your hand rests on the inferior angle of the scapula (figure 2.4). Instruct your client to slowly elevate their arm in the scapular plane.

During the elevation, you will need to mimic the movement of the scapula. Do this by applying pressure upward and laterally to the inferior angle, to facilitate elevation of the scapula, and pull on the superior angle, bringing it backward to simulate posterior tilting of the scapula.

Findings: The test is positive for muscle inhibition if symptoms are reduced during the maneuver.

CHAPTER 3

Supraspinatus

The supraspinatus muscle lies in the supraspinous fossa on the posterior of the scapula and attaches also to the head of the humerus (figure 3.1). Supraspinatus is primarily an abductor of the humerus and is capable of fully abducting the humerus into elevation. This muscle also helps to stabilize the head of the humerus within the glenoid fossa.

The special tests included for supraspinatus are the supraspinatus-specific Painful Arc Test, the Hawkin's-Kennedy Test, the Champagne Toast Test, Jobe's Test (which you may know as the Empty Can Test)—to be contrasted with the Full Can Test, Yocum's Test, the Drop Arm (Codman's) Test, and Neer's Impingement Sign.

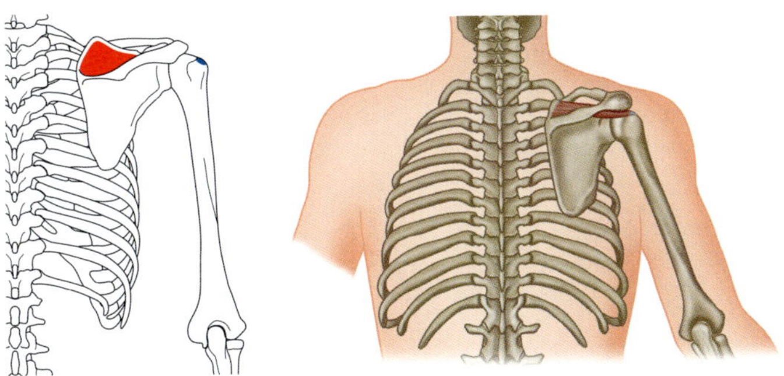

Figure 3.1: The supraspinatus muscle.

Painful Arc Test

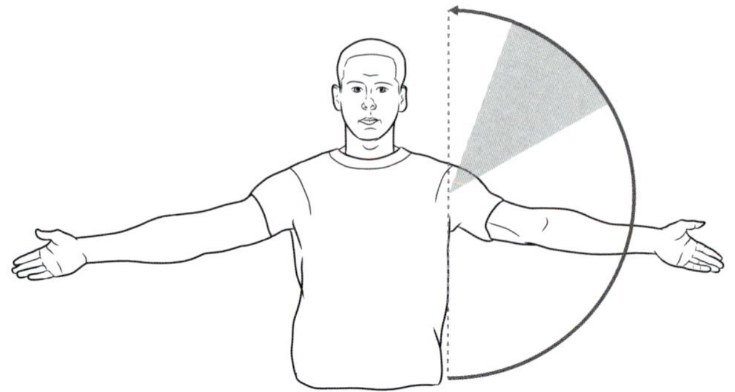

Figure 3.2: Painful Arc Test, showing the 120°–160° arc of pain indicating supraspinatus pathology.

Purpose: This tests for pathology affecting the supraspinatus tendon.

Type of Test: This is an active pain-provocation test. As the test also requires contraction of the shoulder abductor muscles, it tests the strength against gravity of the supraspinatus muscle and the medial fibers of the deltoid muscle.

Procedure: Ensure your client begins with a good, upright sitting or standing posture, as protraction of the scapula affects the test result. Instruct them to abduct the arm through the full ROM.

Findings: Between 160° and 120° of abduction, the supraspinatus tendon is impinged between the acromion and the greater tubercle of the humerus (figure 3.2). Therefore, pain within this range suggests a supraspinatus pathology.

Tip: This test is also used to assess the AC joint, which typically elicits pain in the 140° to 180° range of abduction. Other shoulder pathologies can give rise to a painful arc.

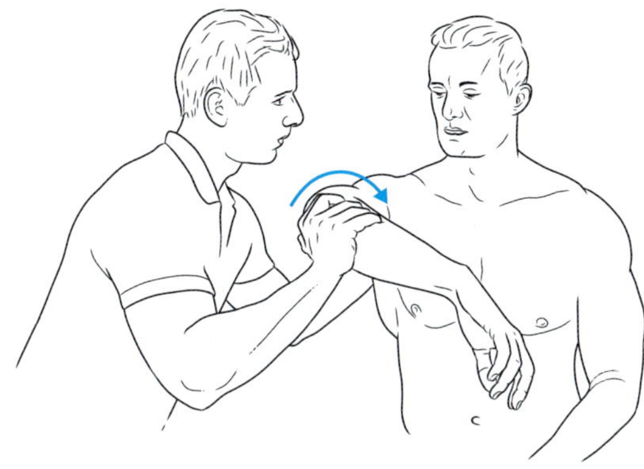

Figure 3.3: Hawkins-Kennedy Test, showing passive internal rotation of the arm with the shoulder and elbow at 90°.

Purpose: Described by Hawkins and Kennedy (1980), this tests for *subacromial impingement* pain.

Type of Test: This is a passive pain-provocation test.

Procedure: With your client seated, passively flex the shoulder and elbow to 90° (figure 3.3). Stabilize the scapula with one hand, and with your other, internally rotate the arm by holding it at the elbow.

Findings: The test is positive if it reproduces the patient's shoulder pain.

Champagne Toast Test

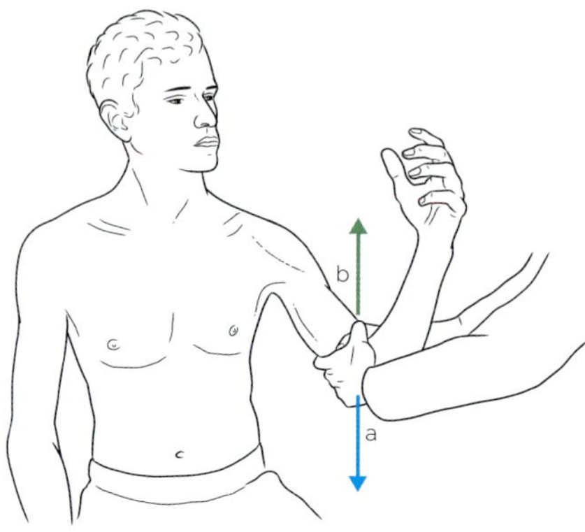

Figure 3.4: Champagne Toast Test, with arrows indicating the direction of force applied by the clinician (a) and the direction of force applied by the client (b).

Purpose: Proposed by Gregory P. Nicholson and described by Chalmers et al. (2016), this tests for pathology of the supraspinatus tendon.

Type of Test: This is a test requiring isometric contraction of the shoulder muscles.

Procedure: Ask your client to raise their arm as if holding a glass to make a toast. In this position the shoulder is in 30° of abduction, 30° of forward flexion, and slight external rotation, plus 90° of elbow flexion. Apply downward pressure to the arm (figure 3.4a) and ask your client to resist this (figure 3.4b), thus performing an isometric contraction.

Findings: The test is positive if it reproduces the client's pain.

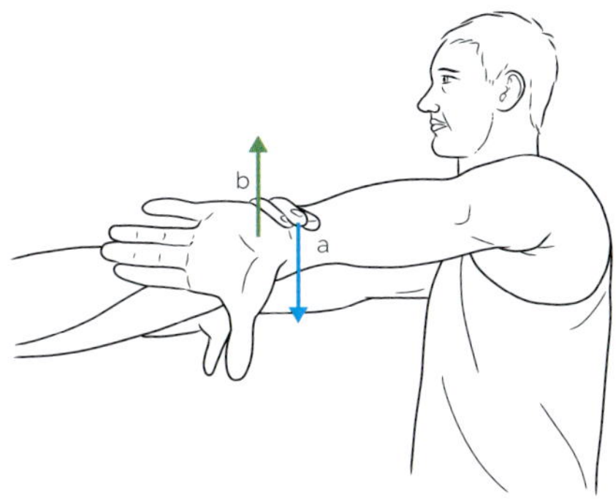

Figure 3.5: Jobe's Test, with arrows indicating the direction of force applied by the clinician (a) and the direction of force applied by the client (b).

Purpose: Described by Jobe and Jobe (1983), this tests for damage and/or weakness to the supraspinatus muscle or tendon.

Type of Test: This is a pain provocation test, which also tests strength of the supraspinatus muscle.

Procedure: Ask your client to adopt the starting position, which mimics emptying a can of liquid: the arms abducted to 90°, around 30°–45° from the midline (the scapular plane), internally rotated so that the thumbs are pointing downward. Apply a downward pressure to the distal forearm (figure 3.5a), asking your client to resist this (figure 3.5b).

Findings: The test is positive if it reproduces the client's pain, or if they are unable to maintain the test position against your downward pressure.

Tip: When applying downward pressure, place your hands close to the wrist where you have greatest leverage, and take care to modify the amount of force you apply depending on your client's physique. For example, a client who performs regular strengthening of the upper limb would require greater pressure than one who does not. The test is often easier for the clinician when performed with the client seated.

Full Can Test

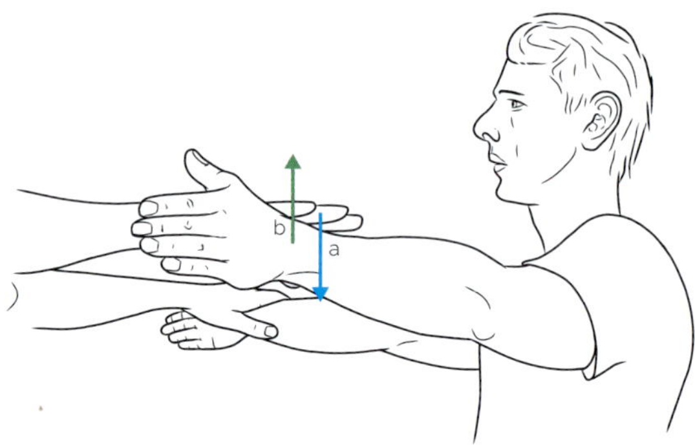

Figure 3.6: Full Can Test, with arrows showing the direction of force applied by the clinician (a) and the direction of force applied by the client (b).

Purpose: Described by Kelly, Kadrmas, and Speer (1996) as the optimal position in which to test the strength of the supraspinatus muscle, this has since been used to test for integrity of the supraspinatus tendon.

Type of Test: This is a muscle strength test, now used also as a pain-provocation test.

Procedure: Ask your client to raise their arms to 90° of flexion in the scapular plane, with thumbs pointing upward. Place downward pressure on the arm (figure 3.6a), and ask your client to resist this (figure 3.6b).

Findings: Supraspinatus tendinopathy is indicated if the test reproduces the client's pain without weakness.

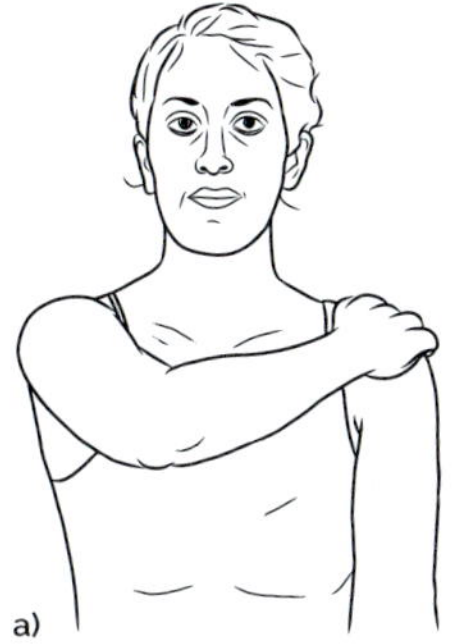

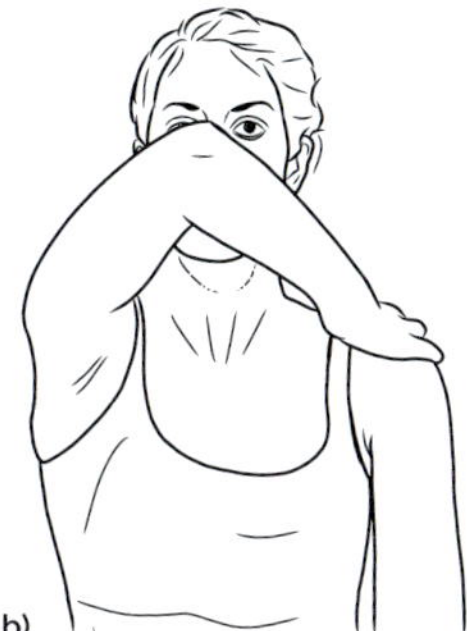

Figure 3.7: Yocum's Test: (a) start position; (b) end position.

Purpose: This tests for subacromial impingement.

Type of Test: This is an active pain-provocation test.

Procedure: With your client sitting or standing, ask them to place the hand of their affected shoulder onto the opposite shoulder (figure 3.7a). In this position, ask the client to elevate the elbow of the affected side (figure 3.7b).

Findings: The test is positive for impingement if there is pain in the region of the subacromial arch.

Drop Arm (Codman's) Test

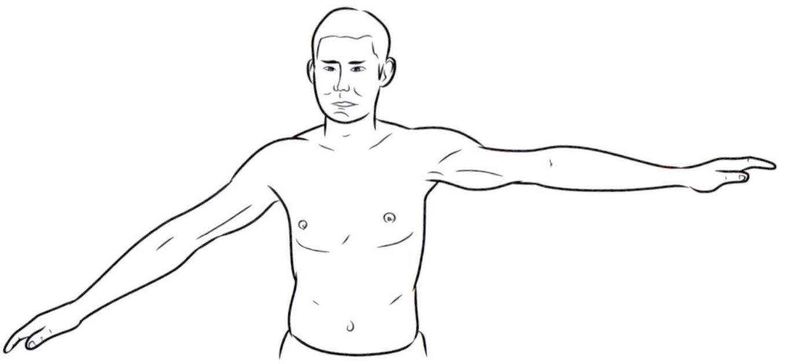

Figure 3.8: A positive Drop Arm (Codman) Test.

Purpose: Described by Codman (1934), this tests for weakness and lesions of supraspinatus. Note that this is different to the Drop Arm Sign described by Hertel et al. (1996).

Type of Test: This is an active test requiring strength in the supraspinatus muscle and the medial fibers of the deltoid muscle.

Procedure: Passively abduct your client's arm to 90°. Remove your support of the arm and ask your client to slowly lower it in a controlled manner.

Findings: The test is positive if the client cannot perform the test and, instead, the arm drops (figure 3.8).

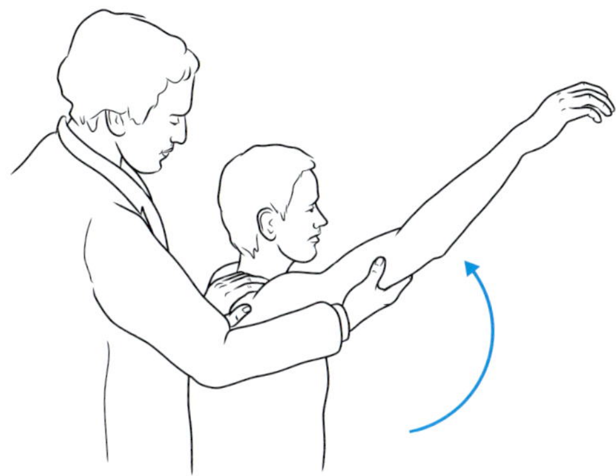

Figure 3.9: Neer's Impingement Sign.

Purpose: Described by Neer (1983), this was designed to test subacromial impingement lesions of the supraspinatus tendon.

The test may also cause pain because of other conditions of the shoulder, such as impingement of the subacromial bursa, the long head of biceps brachii, or other rotator cuff structures.

Type of Test: This is a passive pain-provocation test.

Procedure: With your client seated, stabilize the scapula with one hand, and using your other hand, passively flex your client's arm into elevation (figure 3.9).

Findings: The test is positive for all impingement lesions if the maneuver reproduces the client's pain.

CHAPTER 4

Subscapularis

Subscapularis lies in the subscapular fossa on the anterior surface of the scapula and attaches to the head of the humerus (figure 4.1). Contraction of this muscle primarily brings about medial rotation of the glenohumeral joint. Tests for subscapularis involve medial rotation of the joint with the arm either behind (Gerber's Lift Off Test, Internal Rotation Lag Sign) or in front of the body (Belly Press Test, Napoleon Sign, Belly Off Sign, Bear Hug Test). If you wish to compare the strength of this muscle against that of the lateral rotators of the humerus, please see chapter 5 for the Internal Rotation Resistance Strength Test.

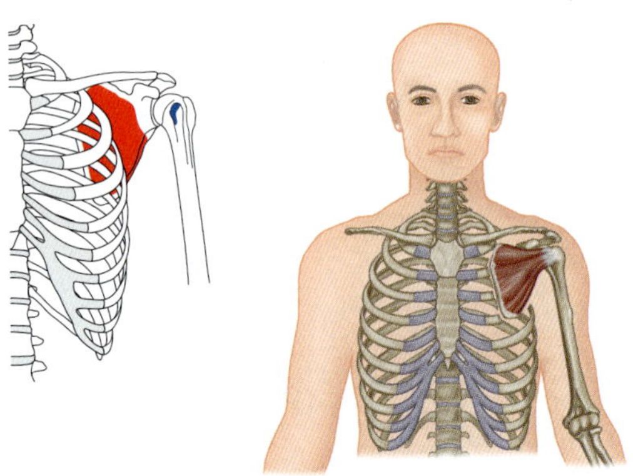

Figure 4.1: The subscapularis muscle.

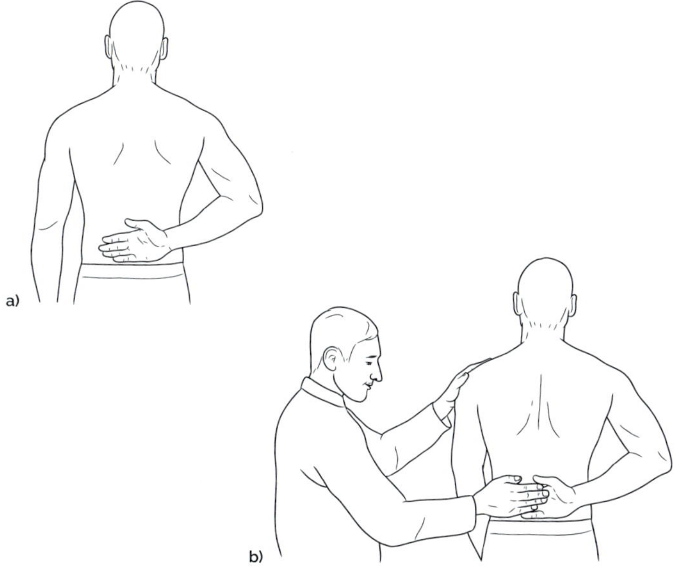

Figure 4.2: Gerber's Lift Off Test: (a) start position; (b) position of the clinician's hand.

Purpose: Described by Gerber and Krushell (1991), this tests for damage and/or weakness in the subscapularis muscle.

Type of Test: This is an active strength test for subscapularis.

Procedure: Ask your client to place the dorsum of their hand on their low back (figure 4.2a) and then to attempt to lift the hand away from the back.

Findings: The test is positive for a lesion in subscapularis if the patient is unable to lift their hand away from their back.

Tip: If your client can take their hand away from their back, you can test the strength of subscapularis by resisting this movement. Place your hand on the client's palm (figure 4.2b), comparing both sides. Differences between the client's ability to lift the right and left hands away from their back can reveal weakness in left and right subscapularis.

Internal Rotation Lag Sign

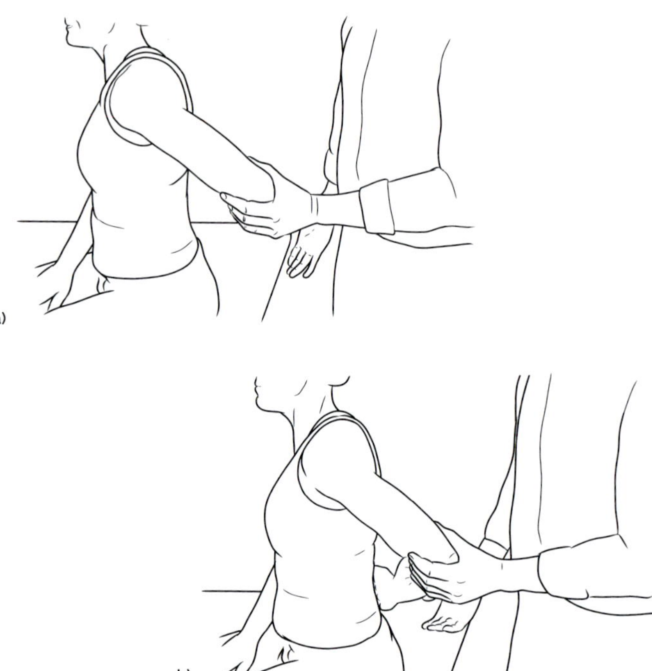

Figure 4.3: Internal Rotation Lag Sign: (a) start position; (b) positive lag sign.

Purpose: Described by Hertel et al. (1996), along with the External Rotation Lag Sign and a test also called the Drop Sign, this tests for full-thickness tears of the subscapularis muscle.

Type of Test: This is an active test of isometric strength in the subscapularis muscle, in which the examiner passively sets the start position.

Procedure: Ask your client to rest the dorsum of their hand on their low back as if for the Gerber Lift Off Test. Holding your client's elbow and wrist, take their arm into 20° of extension (figure 4.3a). In this position, and still holding the elbow, release your client's wrist (figure 4.3b).

Findings: The test is negative if the patient can retain the position (figure 4.3a) and positive for a subscapularis lesion if the wrist drops away from the start position (figure 4.3b).

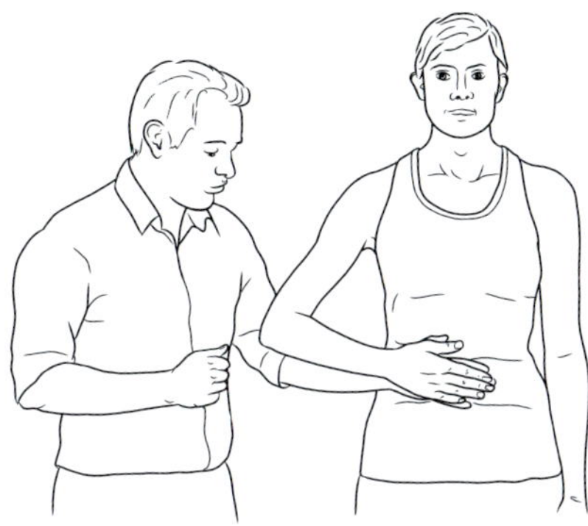

Figure 4.4: Belly Press Test.

Purpose: Described by Gerber, Hersche, and Farron (1996), this tests for integrity of the subscapularis muscle.

Type of Test: This is an active test of strength in the subscapularis muscle.

Procedure: Place the dorsum of your hand against the client's abdomen. Ask your client to place the palm of their hand onto the palm of yours, causing their elbow to flex to around 90° and the arm to internally rotate (figure 4.4). The client should avoid flexion or extension of the wrist, maintaining a neutral wrist position as far as is possible. The client then presses their hand against yours, whilst drawing their elbow forward.

Findings: The test is positive if there is pain and/or the client is unable to perform the test, as pressing into the belly in this position requires internal rotation of the arm, brought about by subscapularis.

Tip: This test may be a useful alternative when restrictions in the client's ability to internally rotate the shoulder rotation limit use of the Gerber's Lift Off Test.

Napoleon Sign

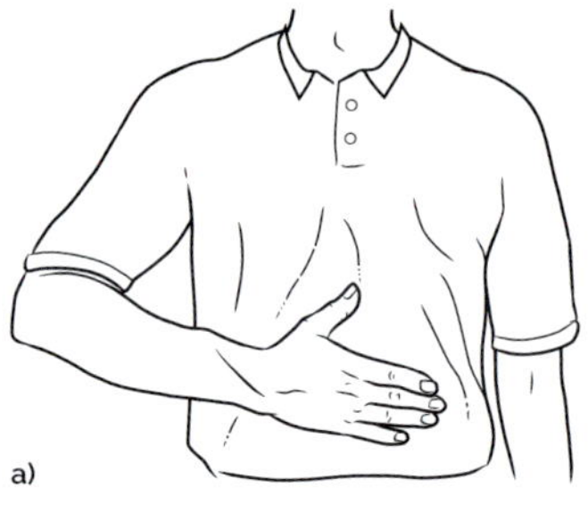

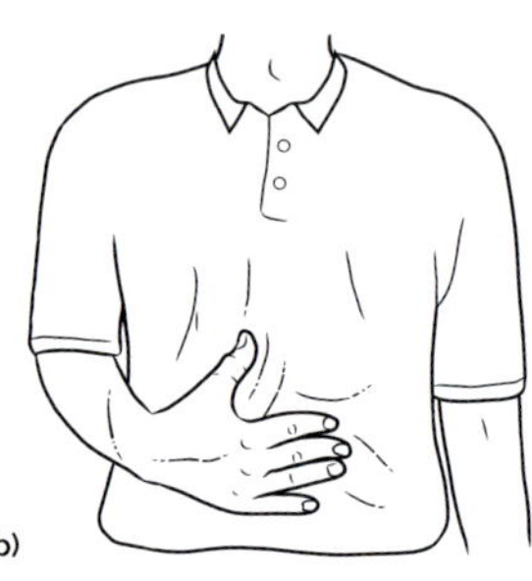

Figure 4.5: Napoleon Sign: (a) start position, with the arm abducted and the wrist in a neutral position; (b) a positive test, showing the arm adducted and the wrist flexed.

Purpose: This is a variant of Gerber's Belly Press Test, and tests for subscapularis integrity.

Type of Test: This is an active test of strength in the subscapularis muscle.

Procedure: The client presses the palm of their hand into their belly, keeping the wrist in neutral, with the elbow out to the side (figure 4.5a).

Findings: The test is positive if the patient cannot retain the wrist in a neutral position but instead the wrist flexes, causing the arm to be brought closer to the side of the body (figure 4.5b).

Tip: Performing the test bilaterally makes comparison between left and right shoulders easier.

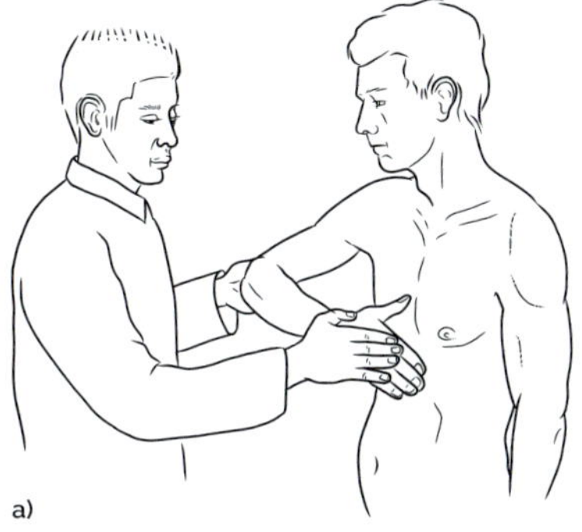

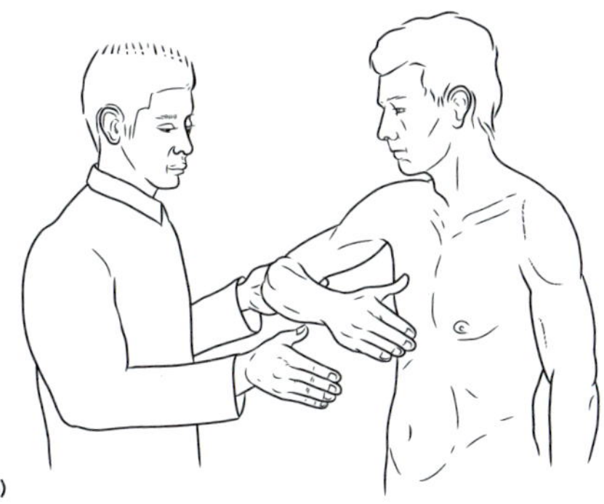

Figure 4.6: Belly Off Sign: (a) start position; (b) a positive test.

Purpose: Described by Scheibel et al. (2005), this tests for lesions of the subscapularis muscle.

Type of Test: This is a test of strength in the subscapularis muscle.

Procedure: The start position is with the client's elbow passively flexed to about 90° and their hand held by you against their abdomen (figure 4.6a). In this position the arm is internally rotated. Whilst maintaining the position of your client's elbow, remove your hand from over the hand of the client that is against their belly.

Findings: The test is positive if the patient cannot retain their hand in the start position against their belly, and it instead moves away from the body slightly (figure 4.6b).

Bear Hug Test

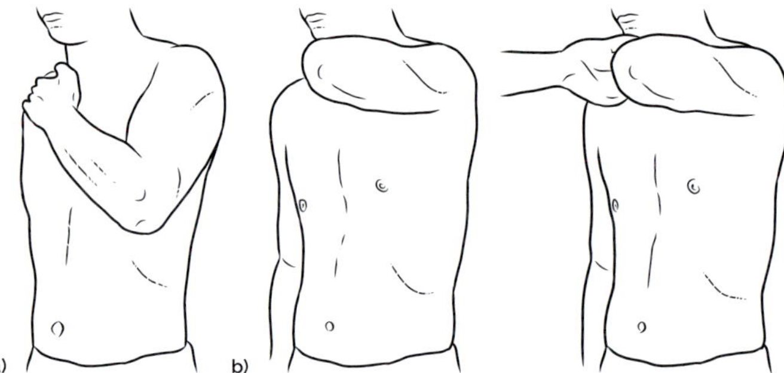

Figure 4.7: Bear Hug Test of the left shoulder, showing the client's hand position on their right shoulder (a) and position of their elbow when performing the test (b).

Figure 4.8: Bear Hug Test, with clinician attempting to remove the client's hand from their shoulder and the client resisting this.

Purpose: Described by Barth, Burkhart, and De Beer (2006), this tests for lesions in the subscapularis muscle.

Type of Test: This is a test of strength in the subscapularis muscle.

Procedure: For the start position your client rests the hand of their affected shoulder on the opposite shoulder (figure 4.7a) with fingers extended. The elbow is then raised so that it is facing forward (figure 4.7b). In this position the arm is internally rotated. Maintaining the position of the elbow, ask your client to press their hand into their shoulder. This requires internal rotation of the arm and thus contraction of subscapularis. Alternatively, as the client maintains the same test position, gently attempt to lift their hand from their shoulder (figure 4.8) and instruct them to resist this. The resistance by the client again requires internal rotation of the arm and thus contraction of subscapularis.

Findings: The test is positive if there is pain and/or the patient cannot retain the start position.

CHAPTER 5

Infraspinatus and Teres Minor

Infraspinatus and teres minor originate on the posterior surface of the scapula and insert onto the head of the humerus (figure 5.1). Both muscles bring about adduction, and their primary action is lateral rotation of the glenohumeral joint. Therefore, an inability to hold the arm in a position of abduction and lateral rotation or difficulty performing a concentric or isometric contraction of the muscles indicates a problem.

This chapter provides information about three tests in which the client is required to hold their arm in abduction and external rotation (External Rotation Lag Sign, Hertel's Drop Sign, Walch's Hornblower Sign), one test that requires the client to perform concentric contraction of the muscles (Patte's Test), and one that requires isometric muscle contraction (Internal Rotation Resistance Strength Test). As the name implies, the Internal Rotation Resistance Strength Test, also tests internal rotation.

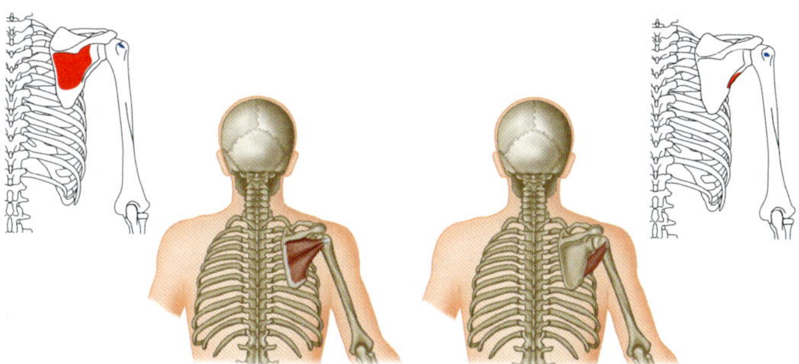

Figure 5.1: Infraspinatus and teres minor muscles.

External Rotation Lag Sign

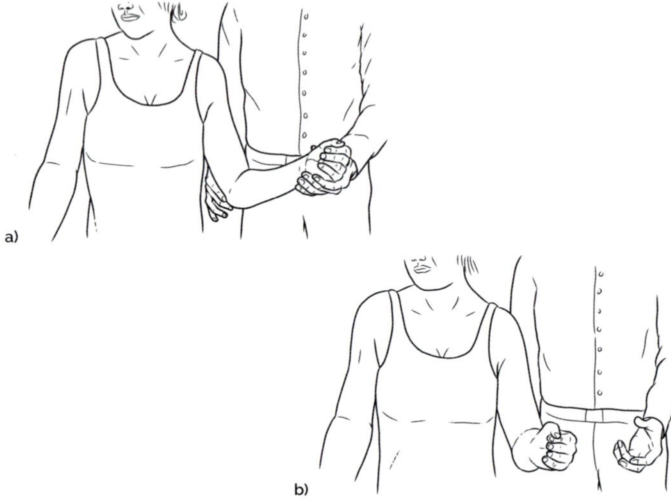

Figure 5.2: External Rotation Lag Sign: (a) start position; (b) a positive lag sign.

Purpose: Described by Hertel et al. (1996), along with the Internal Rotation Lag Sign and (Hertel's) Drop Sign, this tests for rupture predominantly of the infraspinatus and supraspinatus tendons. It has been included here as it specifically requires active contraction of infraspinatus.

Type of Test: This is a test of strength in the lateral rotators of the humerus.

Procedure: With the client's arm by their side, the elbow flexed to approximately 90°, passively elevate the shoulder to about 20° in the scapular plane. Holding the client's forearm at the wrist and elbow, passively place the arm into full external rotation minus 5° (figure 5.2a). Maintaining your support of their elbow, ask your client to maintain this position when you remove your support of their wrist.

Findings: The test is positive if the client cannot retain the position and the arm drifts inward (figure 5.2b). The amount of "lag" can be measured in degrees.

Tip: It is important not to position the arm into full external rotation at the start of the test to minimize the naturally occurring elastic recoil of the joint.

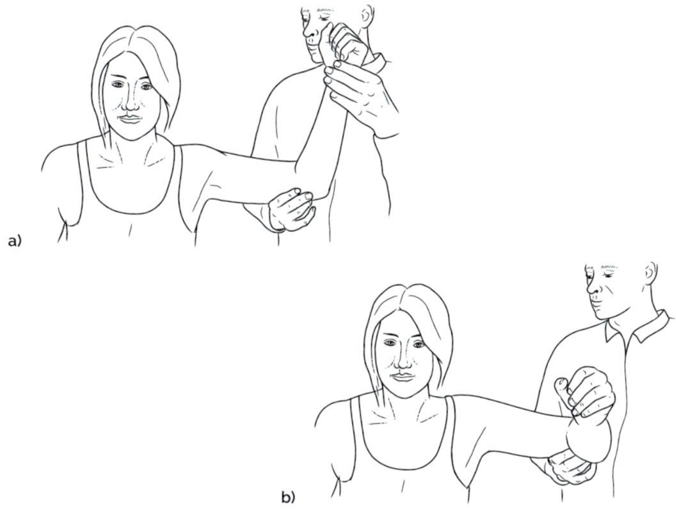

Figure 5.3: Hertel's Drop Sign: (a) start position; (b) a positive test.

Purpose: Described by Hertel et al. (1996), along with the External Rotation Lag Sign and Internal Rotation Lag Sign, this tests for lesions of the infraspinatus. Note that this is different to the Drop Test described by Codman (1934).

Type of Test: This is a test of strength for infraspinatus.

Procedure: With your client's elbow flexed, passively elevate the shoulder to 90°, and almost fully externally rotate the arm with the elbow flexed to 90° (figure 5.3a). Maintaining support of the elbow, ask the client to maintain this position whilst you release their wrist.

Findings: The test is positive if the client is unable to maintain the position (figure 5.3b).

Walch's Hornblower Sign

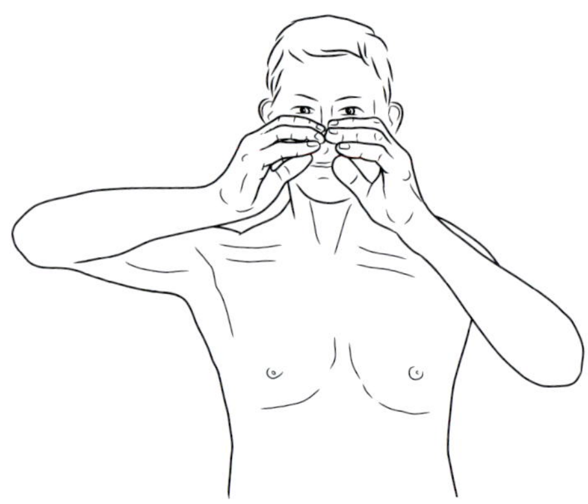

Figure 5.4: Walch's Hornblower Sign, showing a positive test result for the right shoulder.

Purpose: Described by Walch et al. (1998), this test is for pathology affecting teres minor and infraspinatus.

Type of Test: This is a test of strength for the teres minor and infraspinatus muscles.

Procedure: Ask your client to bring both hands to their mouth as if playing a wind instrument such as a horn.

Findings: The test is positive if in order to perform the maneuver the patient has to abduct the affected arm (figure 5.4).

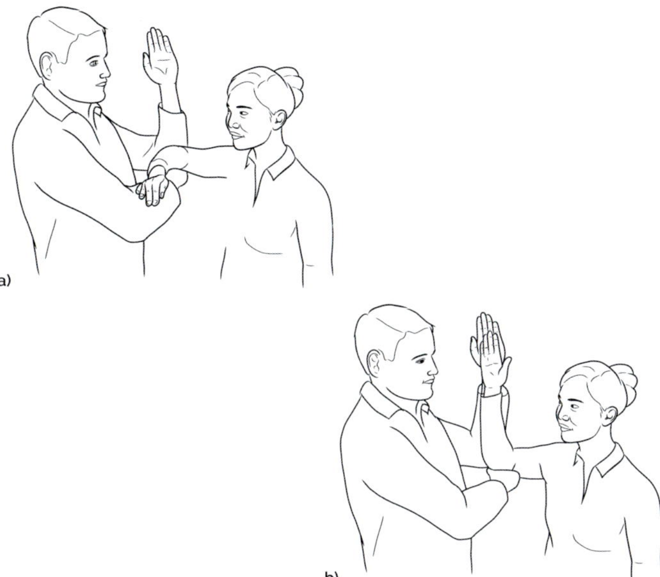

Figure 5.5: Patte's Test: (a) start position; (b) with client performing active isometric contraction of the lateral rotators of the shoulder.

Purpose: Described by Patte and Gerber (1987), this tests for the integrity of the teres minor muscle in the case of a deficient infraspinatus.

Type of Test: This is a strength test, testing the ability of the external shoulder rotators to contract concentrically in order to externally rotate the arm.

Procedure: Begin with your client's arm at 90° of abduction in the scapular plane, with 90° of elbow flexion, using one of your arms to support the client's forearm (figure 5.5a). From this position, ask the client to perform active external rotation of the shoulder against resistance provided by you (figure 5.5b).

Findings: The test is positive if the strength of external rotation is deemed less than Grade 4 as defined by the Medical Research Council (No 1976, 1).

Tip: Another way to support the client's arm is to have them seated at the edge of a table or treatment plinth, the arm supported by blocks or pillows, resting in the start position.

Internal Rotation Resistance Strength Test

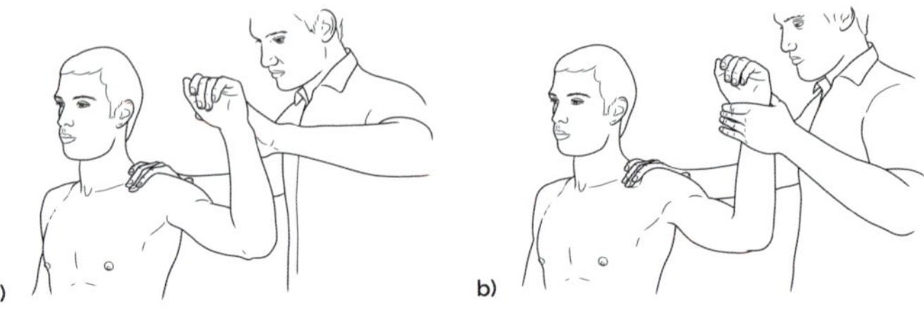

Figure 5.6: Internal Rotation Resistance Strength Test: (a) with client resisting external rotation; (b) with client resisting internal rotation.

Purpose: Described by Zaslav (2001), the Internal Rotation Resistance Strength Test (IRRST) is used to differentiate between intra-articular (within the joint) pathology and impingement of the supraspinatus tendon when this has been indicated by a positive Neer's Impingement Sign (table 5.1). Impingement of the supraspinatus tendon is an example of an extra-articular (outside of the joint) pathology. For details of how to perform the Neer's Impingement Sign test, see page 33.

Type of Test: This is a strength test, comparing the isometric strength of the external shoulder rotators with the isometric strength of the internal shoulder rotators.

Procedure: The test is performed when someone has been assessed to have a positive Neer's Impingement Sign. Passively abduct your client's arm to 90° with 80° of external rotation, with the elbow flexed. Ask your client to maximally resist external rotation (figure 5.6a) and then internal rotation (figure 5.6b) against your pressure.

Findings: The test is positive if the client has good strength in the external position (figure 5.6a) but weakness when internal rotation is performed (figure 5.6b).

Table 5.1: Possible outcomes for the IRRST in someone with a positive Neer's Impingement Sign.

Strength Differences	Pathology Indicated
Strength appears greater in external rotation compared with internal rotation	Intra-articular
Strength appears weaker in external rotation compared with internal rotation	Extra-articular, as in impingement of the supraspinatus tendon proposed by Neer

CHAPTER 6

Labrum of the Glenohumeral Joint

The shoulder joint facilitates a great range of arm movement but is an unstable joint owing to the shallow surface of the scapula (the glenoid fossa) with which the head of the humerus articulates. A rim of cartilage known as the *labrum* helps provide a slightly larger surface area for the head of the humerus, and around this there is a thin joint capsule. Tendons of the many shoulder muscles, as well as ligaments, blend with this capsule to provide reinforcement of the joint (figure 6.1).

Tears of the labrum are common. Superior labrum anterior and posterior tears, known as SLAP lesions, were categorized into four types by Snyder in 1990 (table 6.1). Ahsan, Hsu, and Gee (2016) remind us that multiple subclassifications have since been proposed, and that use of the Synder classification is "widely variable

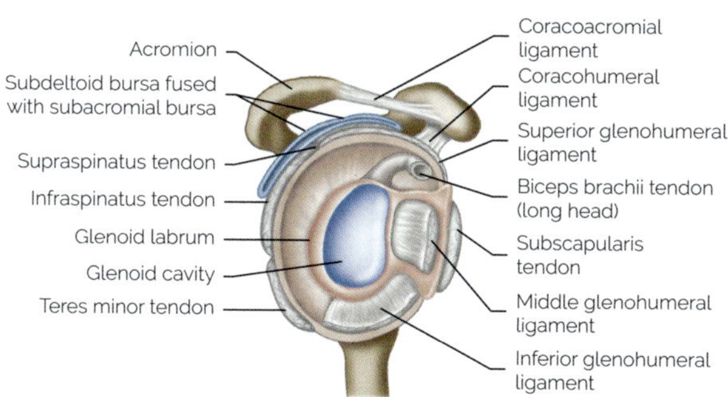

Figure 6.1: The labrum of the right shoulder joint, showing the surrounding ligaments and tendons.

and inconsistent" (p. 2075). Nevertheless, Synder's original four classifications provide a useful starting point to understand the types and severity of lesion that affect the labrum.

Information within this chapter will help you to assess SLAP lesions using Habermeyer's Supine Flexion Resistance Test, the Crank Test (also called the Compression Rotation Test), the Clunk Test, and Kim's Test. The tendon of the long head of biceps brachii is a particularly important structure as it serves to compress the head of the humerus against the glenoid cavity during contraction of the muscle. This tendon courses within the capsule of the shoulder joint and is often damaged in SLAP lesions. Therefore, five special tests for biceps are also included in this chapter. Two of these (Biceps Load Test 1 and Biceps Load Test 2) are designed to test the muscle, and three are aimed specifically at testing the long tendon (Yergason's Test, Speed's Test, Ludington's Test).

Table 6.1: Types of SLAP lesions.

Type	Labral Changes	Biceps Tendon Changes
Type I	Degenerative fraying of the superior labrum; the peripheral labral attachment remains stable	The biceps tendon remains intact and stable
Type II	Degenerative fraying of the superior labrum; detachment of the superior labrum from the glenoid	Detachment of the biceps anchor from the supraglenoid tubercle
Type III	A bucket-hand tear of the superior labrum	The biceps tendon anchor remains intact
Type IV	A bucket-hand tear of the superior labrum	The tear extends into the anchor of the biceps tendon

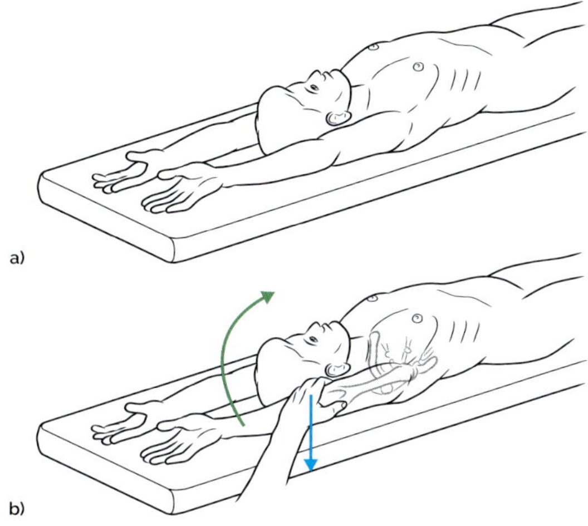

Figure 6.2: Habermeyer's Supine Flexion Resistance Test: (a) start position; (b) position of the clinician's hand distal to the elbow.

Purpose: Attributed to Peter Habermeyer and described by Ebinger et al. (2008), this tests for superior labrum anterior-posterior (SLAP) lesions.

Type of Test: This is a pain-provocation test that requires isometric contraction of the shoulder flexors.

Procedure: The client rests in the supine position with the arms in full elevation, palms upward (figure 6.2a). Ask them to flex their arm, as in a throwing motion, whilst you provide resistance, holding the arm just distal to the elbow (figure 6.2b).

Findings: The test is positive only if there is pain deep inside the shoulder joint or along the joint line.

Crank (Compression Rotation) Test

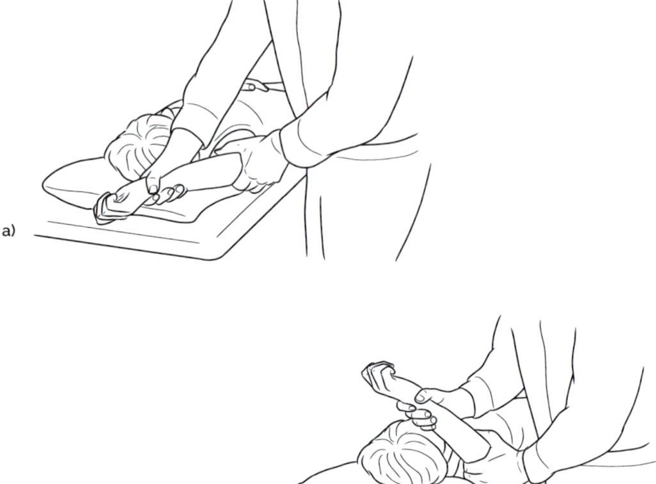

Figure 6.3: Crank Test/Compression Rotation Test: position of the clinician's hands on the client's forearm as the client's arm is taken into external rotation (a) and internal rotation (b).

Purpose: This tests for SLAP lesions.

Type of Test: This is a passive pain-provocation test.

Procedure: Holding your client's forearm, elevate the shoulder into the scapular plane. Apply gentle pressure through the humerus, toward the shoulder, whilst simultaneously externally rotating the shoulder (figure 6.3a). Maintaining pressure through the humerus, internally rotate the shoulder (figure 6.3b).

Findings: The test is positive if there is catching, clicking, and/or pain.

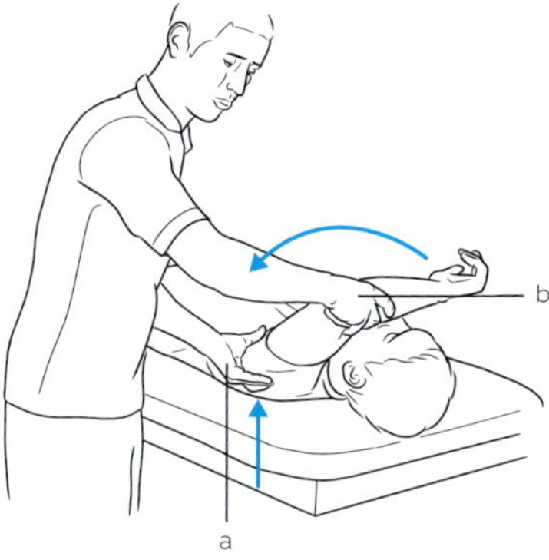

Figure 6.4: The Clunk Test.

Purpose: This tests for SLAP lesions.

Type of Test: This is a passive provocation test that elicits a "clunk" sound.

Procedure: Position your client in supine, with their shoulder slightly over the side of the treatment plinth. Place one of your hands on the posterior of the glenohumeral joint (figure 6.4a), and with your other hand grasp the bicondylar aspect of the humerus above the elbow (figure 6.4b). Next, slowly abduct the arm whilst externally rotating the arm and pushing anteriorly on the humeral head.

Findings: The test is positive for a labral tear if there is a "clunk" sound.

Tip: Snapping, catching, or grinding sensations are all also indicative of a labral tear.

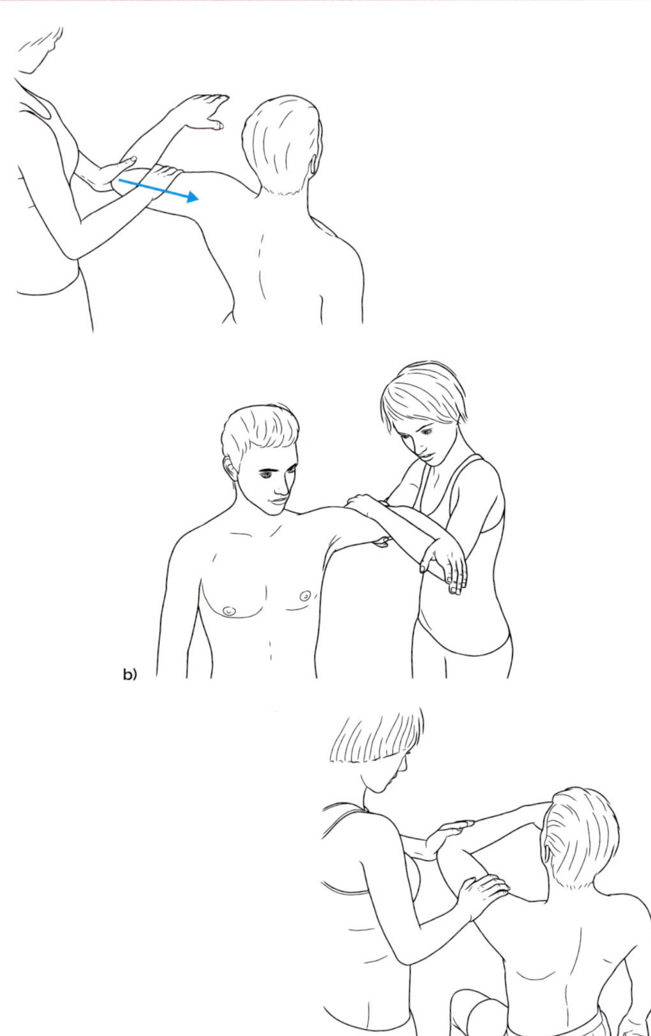

Figure 6.5: Kim's Test: (a) and (b) alternative start positions in which to apply longitudinal force through the humerus; (c) position of the client's arm as it is moved diagonally across the body.

Purpose: Described by Kim et al. (2005), this tests for a posterior-inferior lesion of the glenohumeral labrum.

Type of Test: This is a passive pain-provocation test.

Procedure: Support your client's arm in 90° of abduction and apply a longitudinal force through the humerus (figure 6.5a). In the original research, Kim illustrates the examiner applying the axial load using their hand. You may, however, find it more comfortable to apply the axial load by resting the client's flexed elbow against your body as shown here (figure 6.5b). The arm is then moved across the body, diagonally upward to 45°, with both an inferior and a posterior force applied to the proximal arm (figure 6.5c), whilst also maintaining the axial pressure.

Findings: The test is positive for a posterior-inferior lesion if there is sudden onset posterior shoulder pain.

Tip: Kim notes that it is important for the client to counter the axial loading of the arm, and they should therefore sit on a chair with a back rather than on a stool.

Biceps Load Test 1

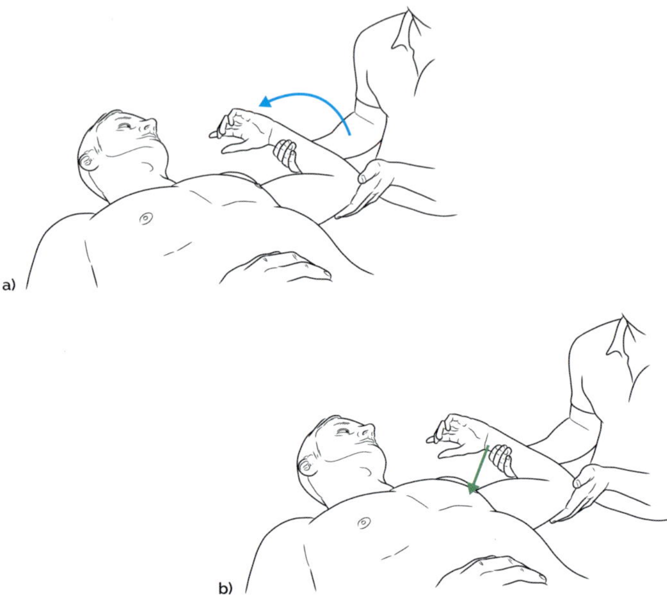

Figure 6.6: Biceps Load Test 1: (a) start position of the shoulder apprehension test with the arm in external rotation; (b) isometric elbow flexion.

Purpose: This tests for SLAP lesions in people with anterior shoulder instability.

Type of Test: This is a passive pain-provocation test.

Procedure: The client is in the supine position. Perform a shoulder apprehension test first: Passively abduct the arm to 90°, with the elbow flexed to 90° and the forearm supinated, then slowly externally rotate the arm (figure 6.6a). Stop external rotation at the point where your client appears apprehensive. At this point, ask your client to flex the elbow against resistance (figure 6.6b). Ask them whether flexing the elbow against resistance in this position increases the apprehension they feel or whether it worsens the pain.

Findings: The test is positive if there is no change in the amount of apprehension felt by the client or if the shoulder becomes more painful. If pain or apprehension are reduced, the test is negative.

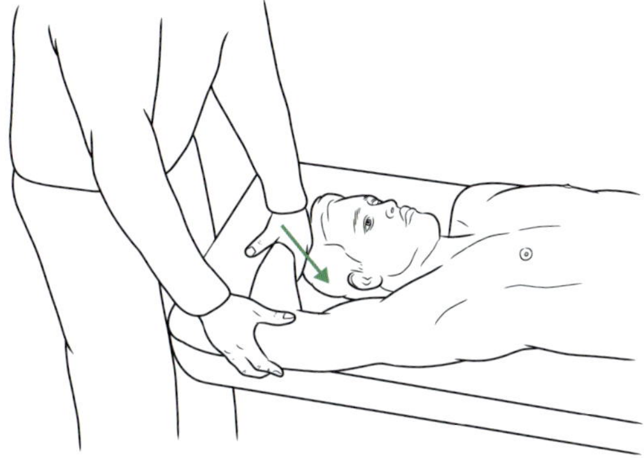

Figure 6.7: Biceps Load Test 2, position with isometric elbow flexion.

Purpose: This tests for SLAP lesions.

Type of Test: This is a passive pain-provocation test involving isometric contraction of biceps brachii.

Procedure: With the client in the supine position, take their arm passively into 120° of elevation and external rotation, with the elbow flexed to 90°. The client is then instructed to flex the elbow against resistance (figure 6.7).

Findings: The test is positive for a SLAP lesion if there is pain in the joint during resisted elbow flexion.

Yergason's Test

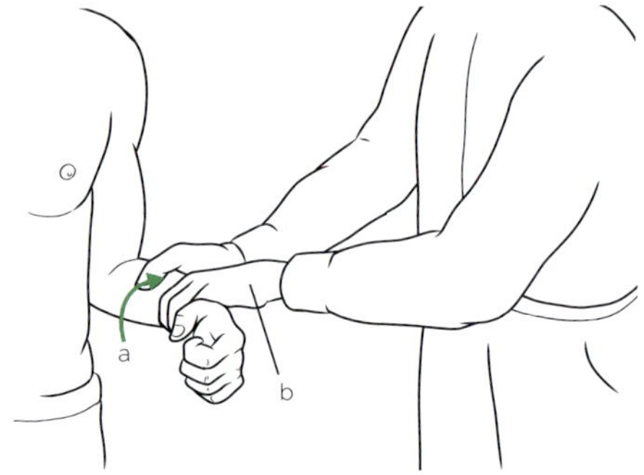

Figure 6.8: Yergason's Test: (a) client performs supination; (b) therapist provides resistance to supination.

Purpose: Described by Yergason (1931) from a single case report, this tests for pathology of the biceps brachii tendon and for a SLAP lesion.

Type of Test: This is a pain-provocation test involving isometric contraction of biceps brachii and supinator muscles.

Procedure: Your client sits or stands with their elbow flexed to 90°, the wrist pronated. Ask them to supinate the wrist/forearm (figure 6.8a) whilst you provide resistance to this (figure 6.8b).

Yergason did not provide an illustration of the therapist's hand position. In my experience, grasping the distal forearm (rather than the wrist) provides adequate leverage against strong clients whilst avoiding strain to their wrist. You should be aware, however, that there is no definitive hand position for this test. Pettitt et al. (2008) provide a useful overview of hand placements for performing the Yergason test in leading textbooks at the time of writing.

Findings: The test is positive if there is pain in the bicipital groove. Clicking in the bicipital groove indicates damage to the transverse humeral ligament, as this would normally retain the biceps tendon in that groove.

Tip: Fibers from the subscapularis tendon may support the biceps tendon, and therefore subscapularis should be tested when Yergason's test is positive for subluxation of the biceps brachii tendon.

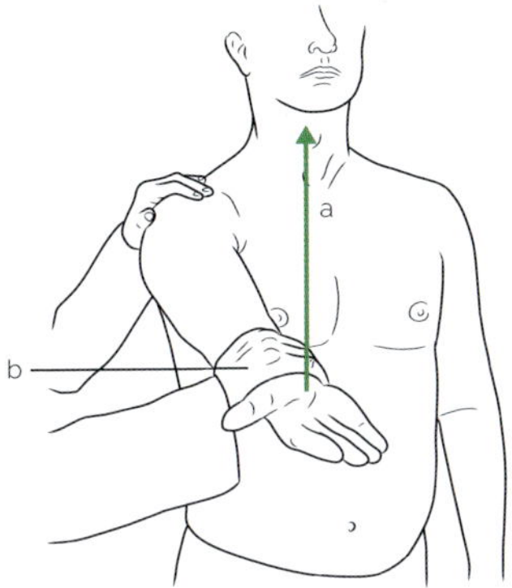

Figure 6.9: Speed's Test, showing the attempted direction of movement of the shoulder by the client (a) and the resistance provided by the therapist (b).

Purpose: Crenshaw and Kilgore (1966) cite a personal communication with Speed as the source of this test for tenosynovitis of the long tendon of biceps brachii.

Type of Test: This is a pain-provocation test.

Procedure: With their elbow extended and forearm supinated, ask your client to flex their shoulder (figure 6.9a) against resistance provided by you (figure 6.9b).

Findings: The test is positive if there is pain localized to the bicipital groove.

Ludington's Test

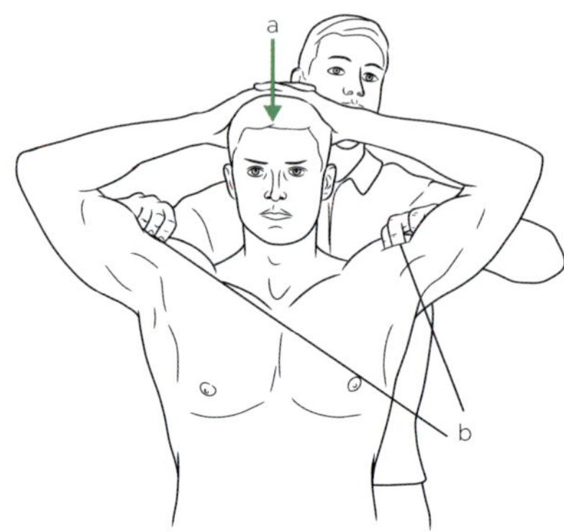

Figure 6.10: Ludington's Test: (a) direction of force applied by the client; (b) hand position of the therapist.

Purpose: Described by Ludington (1923), this tests for proximal biceps brachii tendinopathy or rupture.

Type of Test: This is a test requiring isometric contraction of the biceps brachii muscle.

Procedure: With your client seated with their hands resting palm-down on their head, fingers interlocked to support the weight of the arms, ask them to press down onto their head (figure 6.10a, green arrow) whilst you simultaneously palpate the long head of the biceps brachii tendon bilaterally using two fingers (figure 6.10b).

Findings: The test is positive for a rupture of the long head of the biceps brachii tendon when contraction of the tendon is absent and when there is a visible "Popeye" deformity.

CHAPTER 7

Shoulder Instability

As described in chapter 6, the shoulder provides a wide range of arm movement but lacks stability. Gerber and Nyffeler (2002) offer a useful classification of glenohumeral instability (see table 7.1), roughly grouping types of instability into three classes.

Class A instabilities: These are static instabilities. The humeral head is displaced and fixed in a superior, anterior, or posterior position relative to its normal position in the glenoid fossa. Classic symptoms of instability are absent. The diagnosis of instability is made using radiologic findings not clinical findings.

Class B instabilities: These are dynamic instabilities. There is a subjective loss of normal glenohumeral joint stability. There is a momentary loss of joint congruity, but this can be restored. Such instabilities are always initiated by trauma, either repetitive microtrauma or a single traumatic event.

Class C instabilities: People within this class of instability can dislocate their shoulder at will.

Table 7.1: Classification of shoulder instability.

Class	Description	Signs
A1	Static superior subluxation	Nil
A2	Static anterior subluxation	Nil
A3	Static posterior subluxation	Nil
A4	Static inferior subluxation	Nil
B1	Chronic, locked dislocation of the shoulder	Caused by major trauma; the special tests described in this text are not used as there may be fracture present
B2	Unidirectional instability without hyperlaxity	• No sulcus sign • Negative anterior and posterior drawer tests • A positive apprehension test either anterior or posterior • In anterior instability the Gagey (2001) hyperabduction test is positive
B3	Unidirectional instability with hyperlaxity	• Sulcus sign present • A positive anterior *or* a positive posterior apprehension test, not both • Positive anterior drawer test • Positive posterior drawer test • Anterior instability—positive hyperabduction test • Posterior instability—internal rotation of the 90° abducted arm is increased compared with the asymptomatic side
B4	Multidirectional instability without hyperlaxity	• No sulcus sign • Positive anterior apprehension test • Positive posterior apprehension test • External rotation of the adducted arm is not beyond 70° • Negative drawer tests
B5	Multidirectional instability with hyperlaxity	• Positive anterior, posterior, and inferior drawer tests with apprehension in at least two directions • Internal rotation is increased markedly from normal • External rotation is increased markedly from normal

Table 7.1: (continued)

Class	Description
C	There are three groups of people within this category: • Those who can dislocate and relocate their shoulder at will and have control over the placement of the shoulder whether this is within or without the glenoid fossa (Gerber and Nyffeler argue that this is not instability as there is no loss of control) • Those who experience dynamic instability; they learn to subluxate and then reduce the joint • Those who voluntarily subluxate the joint to gain attention or to mask a psychiatric problem and should be viewed as having a psychiatric illness

Tests of joint stability involve being able to passively displace the humeral head from the glenoid fossa. Gerber and Nyffeler remind us that this alone does not indicate instability but, rather, is an assessment of hyperlaxity; passive translation of the humeral head may be a sign of instability if it differs significantly from the asymptomatic shoulder or is associated with symptoms of apprehension.

In this chapter you will find 11 tests you can use to help determine whether your client has shoulder instability. These are Neer's Test (also known as a sulcus sign), Rowe's Test, the Gagey Hyperabduction Test, the Dugas Test, the Load and Shift Test, the Anterior Instability Apprehension Test, the Anterior Drawer Test, the Fulcrum Test, the Posterior Apprehension Test, the Posterior Drawer Test, and the Jerk Test.

Neer's Test (Sulcus Sign)

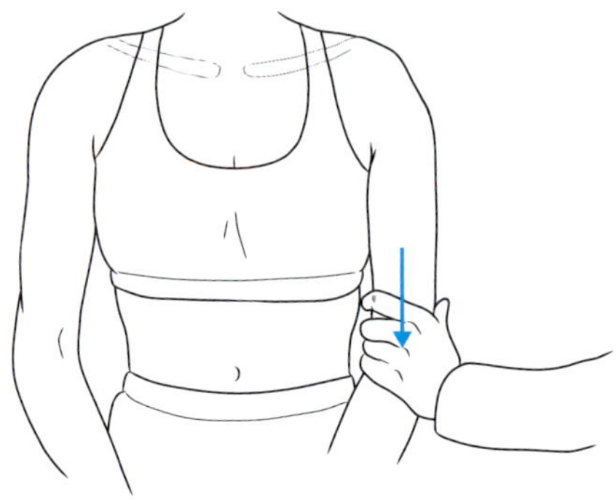

Figure 7.1: Neer's Test (sulcus sign).

Purpose: Described by Neer and Foster (1980), this tests for inferior instability of the glenohumeral joint.

Type of Test: This is a passive traction test.

Procedure: With your client sitting upright and their shoulder muscles relaxed, apply gentle traction to the shoulder by grasping the arm above the elbow (figure 7.1).

Findings: The test is positive if a step-like indentation known as a *sulcus sign* appears on traction of the arm.

Tip: Inferior instability is associated with multidirectional instability and therefore this should not be the only test used to help establish stability of the glenohumeral joint.

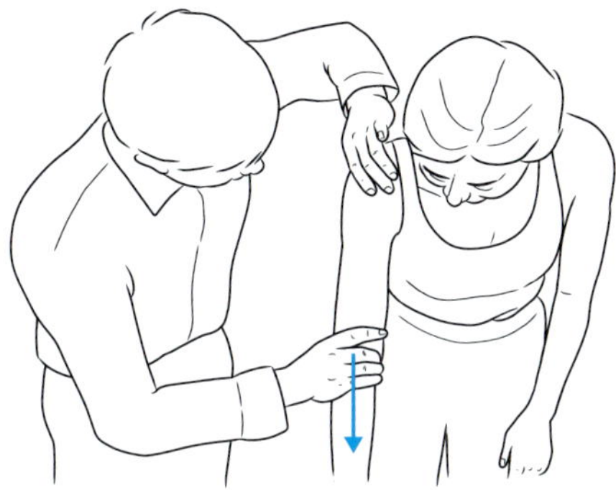

Figure 7.2: Rowe's Test.

Purpose: Described by Rowe, Pierce, and Clark (1973), this tests for inferior subluxation of the shoulder.

Type of Test: This is a passive traction test.

Procedure: With your client standing, ask them to bend forward slightly so that the arm hangs loosely. With the arm in a slightly flexed position, apply gentle traction (figure 7.2).

Findings: The test is positive if a step-like indentation known as a *sulcus sign* appears at the shoulder.

Gagey Hyperabduction Test

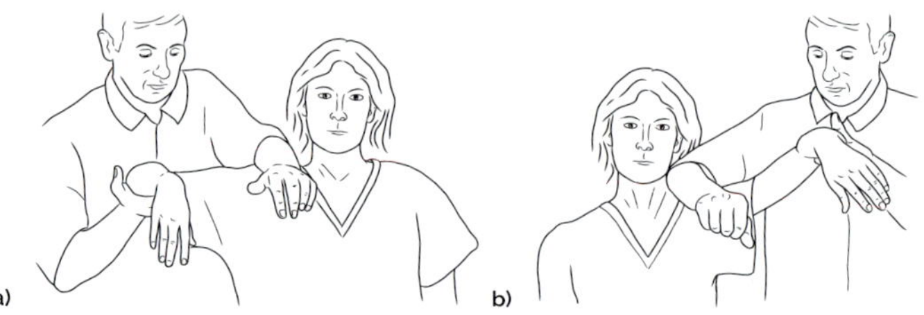

Figure 7.3: Gagey Hyperabduction Test: (a) start position; (b) positive test results.

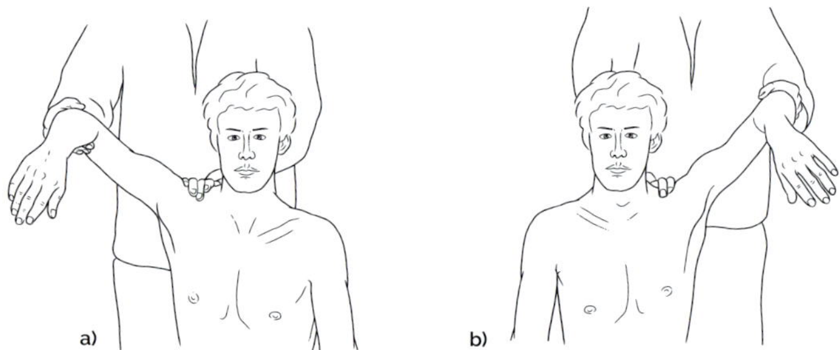

Figure 7.4: Gerber and Nyffeler positive test result evidenced by a 10° difference in abduction of the nonaffected shoulder (a) with the affected shoulder (b).

Purpose: Described by Gagey (2001), this tests for integrity of the inferior glenohumeral ligament.

Type of Test: This is a passive joint movement test.

Procedure: Standing behind your client, gently depress their shoulder girdle passively, using your forearm. Next, abduct the shoulder to 90° (figure 7.3a).

Findings: Gagey reports the test is positive if the clinician can elevate the arm above 90° (figure 7.3b). Gerber and Nyffeler (2002) state that the test is positive if there is a greater than 10° difference in elevation of the nonaffected shoulder (figure 7.4a) with the affected shoulder (figure 7.4b).

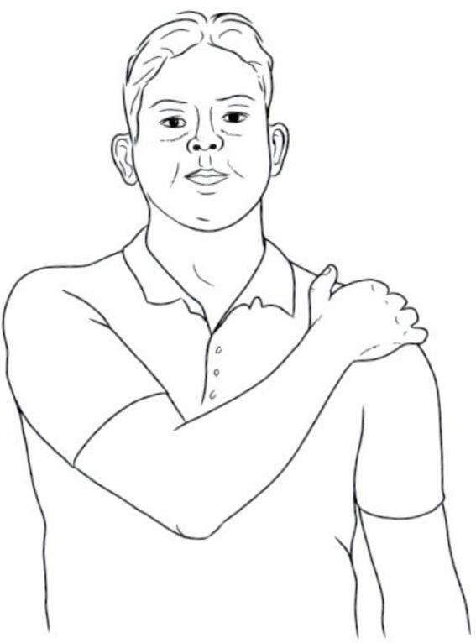

Figure 7. 5: Dugas Test.

Purpose: Reported by Dugas (1857), this tests for anterior dislocation of the glenohumeral joint.

Type of Test: This is an active joint movement test.

Procedure: Ask your client to place the hand of their affected shoulder onto the nonaffected shoulder, then rest the elbow of this arm against their chest (figure 7.5).

Findings: Inability to attain the test position indicates anterior dislocation of the glenohumeral joint.

Load and Shift Test

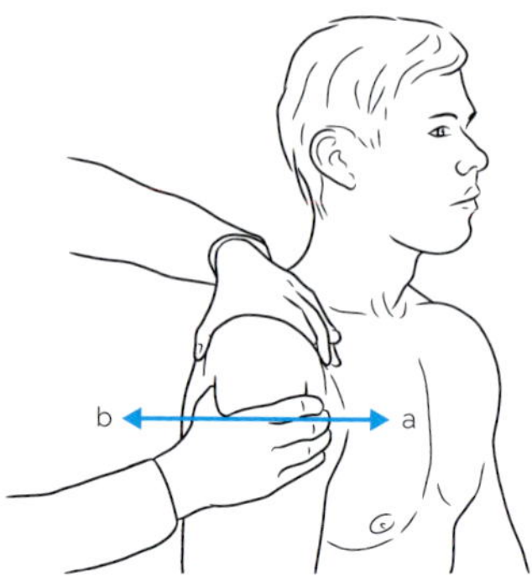

Figure 7.6: Load and Shift Test, with the humeral head pressed anteriorly (a) and posteriorly (b).

Purpose: Described by Silliman and Hawkins (1993), this tests for laxity of the humeral head in the glenohumeral fossa in both an anterior and a posterior direction.

Type of Test: This is a passive joint movement test.

Procedure: The client sits upright with their arm resting on their thigh. The clinician stabilizes the scapula and clavicle with one hand, and with the other hand pinches the humeral head between fingers and thumb. The other shoulder is tested and compared.

- **Load:** The clinician tries to position the humeral head centrally to the glenoid fossa.
- **Shift:** To test the anterior capsule of the joint, the clinician presses the posterior of the humeral head, translating the humeral head anteriorly (figure 7.6a). To test the posterior capsule of the joint, the clinician uses their fingers to translate the humeral head posteriorly (figure 7.6b).

Findings: The test is positive if the affected side translates more than the nonaffected side and reproduces the client's symptoms.

Tip: It does not matter whether the affected or the nonaffected shoulder is tested first. However, many people are apprehensive about movement of the affected joint, so testing the nonaffected side first serves to demonstrate to the client what to expect.

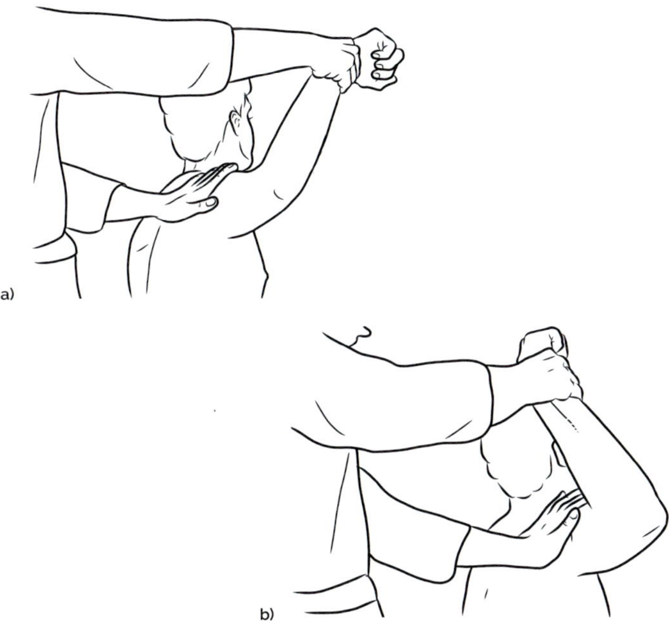

Figure 7.7: Anterior Instability Apprehension Test: (a) beginning of the test with the arm passively abducted to 90°; (b) subsequent external rotation of the arm.

Purpose: This tests for instability of the glenohumeral joint.

Type of Test: This is a passive joint movement test.

Procedure: Flex your client's elbow to 90° and then slowly, passively abduct the shoulder to 90° (figure 7.7a). In this position the arm is then externally rotated (figure 7.7b).

Findings: The test is positive if the client demonstrates apprehension of shoulder dislocation. Apprehension is experienced as a tensing the shoulder muscles in an attempt by the client to counteract movement of the shoulder by the examiner.

Tip: It can be easier to perform the test with the client supine as there is less activation of muscles in this resting position.

Anterior Drawer Test

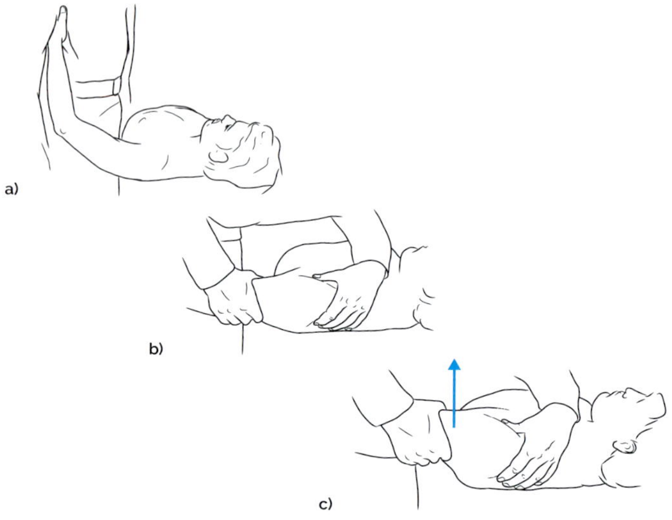

Figure 7.8: Anterior Drawer Test: (a) beginning with the client's hand resting against the axilla of the clinician; (b) the clinician grasps the arm and moves it into 80°–120° abduction, 0°–20° flexion, and 0°–30° lateral rotation; (c) the clinician translates the humeral head anteriorly whilst fixing the scapula.

Purpose: Described by Gerber and Ganz (1984), this tests for instability of the glenohumeral joint, specifically laxity in the anterior shoulder capsule.

Type of Test: This is a passive joint movement test.

Procedure: With your client in the supine position, place their hand beneath the axilla of your arm (figure 7.8a). This helps the client to relax the muscles of the upper limb, making translation of the humeral head easier. Fix the spine of the client's scapula with the fingers of one hand, with the thumb of that hand on the coracoid process. Next, grasp the upper part of the humerus with your other hand, abducting the arm to between 80° and 120°, with 0–20° of flexion, and 0–30° lateral rotation (figure 7.8b). Now translate the humeral head anteriorly whilst fixing the scapula (figure 7.8c).

Findings: The test is positive if there is greater translation of the humeral head of the affected shoulder compared with the nonaffected shoulder.

Tip: Audible clicking may indicate a labral tear, whether or not there is pain.

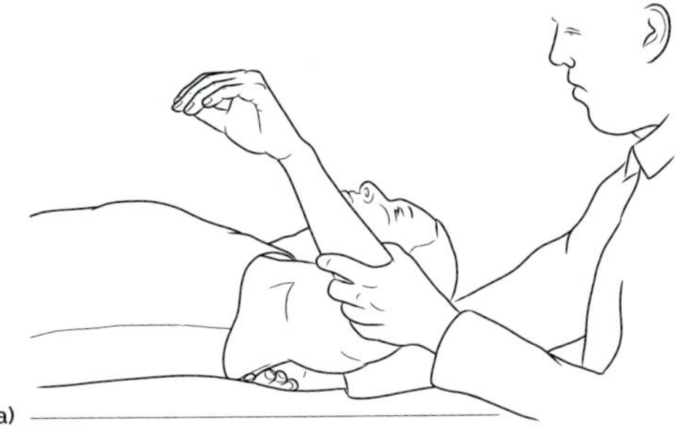

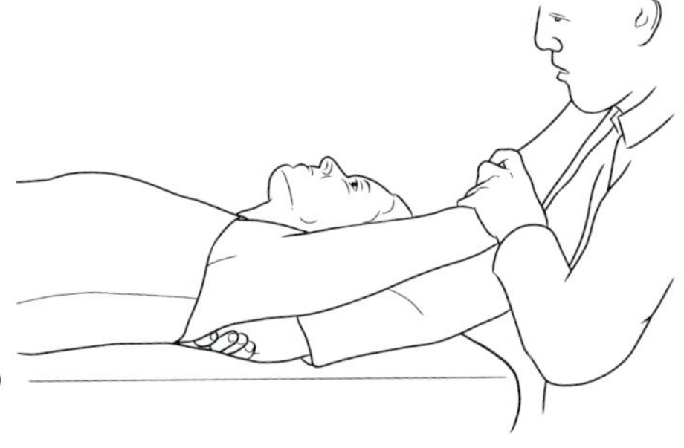

Figure 7.9: Fulcrum Test: (a) beginning with the clinician making a fist, which acts as a fulcrum; (b) the clinician extends and externally rotates the arm over the fulcrum.

Purpose: This tests glenohumeral anterior instability.

Type of Test: This is passive joint movement test.

Procedure: This test is performed with your client in the supine position. Place your hand beneath their shoulder, making a fist, which acts as a fulcrum (figure 7.9a), and grasp the client's forearm, with the elbow flexed to 90°. Next, passively extend and externally rotate the arm over the fulcrum (figure 7.9b).

Findings: The test is positive if there is visible anterior instability of the glenohumeral joint or if the client is apprehensive during this maneuver.

Tip: It can be easier to perform the test by sitting at the head of the treatment plinth, slightly to the side.

Posterior Apprehension Test

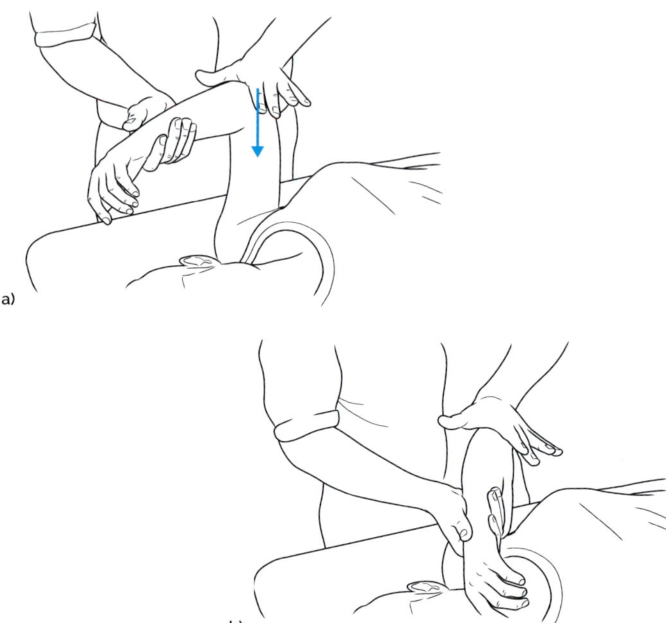

Figure 7.10: Posterior Apprehension Test: (a) beginning with the clinician applying longitudinal pressure through the humerus with the client in the supine position; (b) internally rotating and abducting the arm whilst maintaining the longitudinal pressure.

Purpose: This tests for posterior instability of the glenohumeral joint.

Type of Test: This is a passive joint movement test.

Procedure: Begin with your client in the supine position. With the elbow flexed, passively move the arm into about 90° of flexion, then apply longitudinal pressure through the humerus (figure 7.10a). Next, internally rotate the arm and adduct it whilst maintaining longitudinal pressure through the humerus (figure 7.10b).

Findings: The test is positive if there is apprehension and/or pain in the shoulder at any point during the maneuver.

Tip: Movement of the shoulder is halted if the client appears apprehensive.

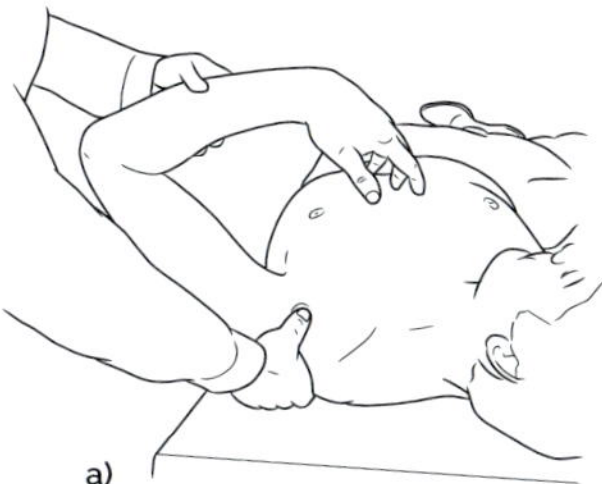

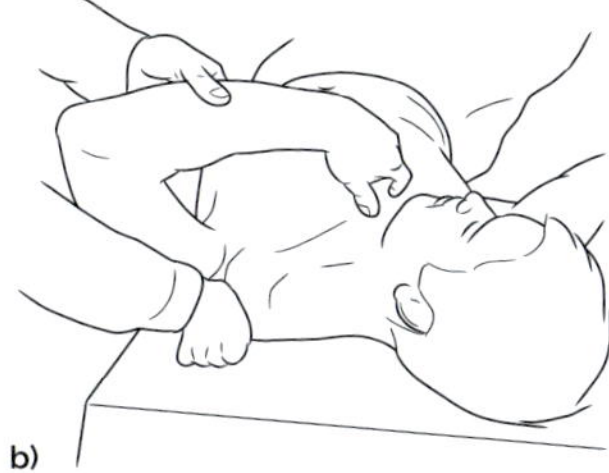

Figure 7.11: Posterior Drawer Test: (a) locate the humeral head whilst the ulnar side of the thumb remains in contact with the lateral aspect of the coracoid; (b) use the thumb to sublux the humeral head posteriorly.

Purpose: This tests for posterior subluxation of the glenohumeral joint. The test illustrated here was described by Gerber and Ganz (1984).

Type of Test: This is a passive joint movement test.

Procedure: To conduct this test, you will press the shoulder posteriorly. Use your hand that is opposite to the shoulder you are testing—when testing the left shoulder, use your right hand to press the shoulder back; when testing the right shoulder, use your left hand. With your client supine, first use one hand to fix the spine of the scapula with your fingers, and locate the coracoid process using your thumb. Use your other hand to position the shoulder whilst holding the client's forearm: the elbow is flexed to about 120°, with the shoulder in 80°–120° of abduction and 20° of flexion.

Now move your thumb slightly lateral to the coracoid process, onto the head of the humerus (figure 7.11a). Gerber and Ganz state that the ulnar side of the thumb should remain in contact with the lateral aspect of the coracoid. The upper arm is then slightly rotated medially and flexed to 60° or 80°.

Whilst performing this maneuver, use your thumb to sublux the humeral head (figure 7.11b). The amount of posterior displacement can be discerned by feeling your thumb glide along the lateral aspect of the coracoid process.

Findings: Although pain-free, the client will often exhibit apprehension. The humeral head will either remain in the glenoid fossa, move back gradually, or sublux. The test is positive if there is subluxation.

Jerk Test

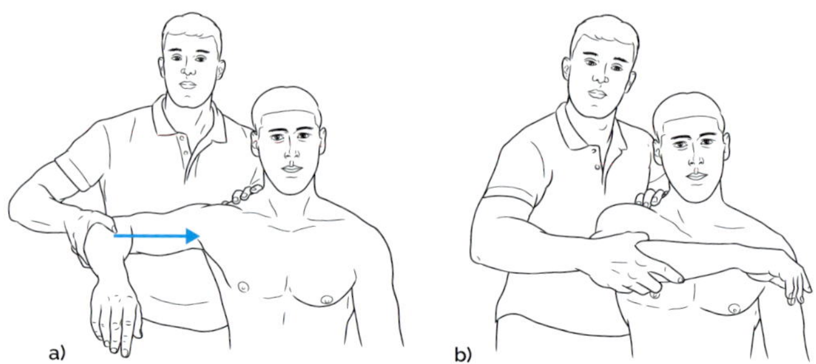

Figure 7.12: The Jerk Test: (a) beginning with passive abduction of the arm to 90°, with the elbow flexed to 90°, then internal rotation of the arm; (b) longitudinal pressure is then applied through the humerus, whilst the arm is moved into horizontal adduction.

Purpose: This tests for posterior instability of the glenohumeral joint. It may be used to test for posterior-inferior labral tears.

Type of Test: This is a passive joint movement test.

Procedure: The test may be performed with the client seated or standing, but it is usually easier for the examiner if the client is seated. Whilst stabilizing the scapula with one hand, passively abduct the arm to 90°, with the elbow flexed to 90°, then internally rotate the arm (figure 7.12a). Then apply longitudinal pressure through the humerus, whilst you move the arm into horizontal adduction (figure 7.12b).

Findings: The test is positive if during the maneuver there is posterior subluxation of the glenohumeral joint accompanied with a "clunk."

Tip: On returning to the start position there is usually a "clunk" as the humeral head is relocated.

PART II

THE ELBOW

The elbow comprises the bones of the humerus, radius, and ulna (figure II.1)—and the joints that these form—and these three bones join in three places. The distal end of the humerus articulates with the proximal end of the ulna to form the humeroulnar joint. This permits the hinge-joint motion of the elbow, with which you may be familiar.

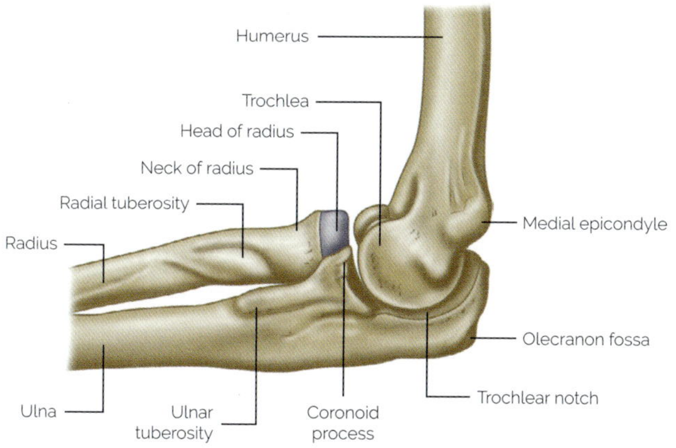

Figure II.1: Right elbow, medial view in 90° flexion.

The humerus also comes into play with the head of the radius at the humeroradial joint. In full extension of the elbow there is no contact between the humerus and radial heads but in flexion the rim of the radius slides into a groove known as the *capitotrochlear groove*. Once the elbow is fully flexed, the radial head makes contact with a special indentation in the humerus called the *radial fossa*. This joint is sometimes called a hinge/pivot joint, owing to the motion it permits.

The radius and ulna are linked also—by the anular ligament—at the proximal radioulnar joint (figure II.2). This is a pivot joint. You can read more about these articulations in chapter 9, "Stability Tests."

In this part of the book you will find 18 tests, not only for the common conditions of medial and lateral epicondylalgia (chapter 8), but also to help you assess the stability of the elbow (chapter 9) and whether there may be any nerve compression (chapter 10) or soft tissue pathology (chapter 11).

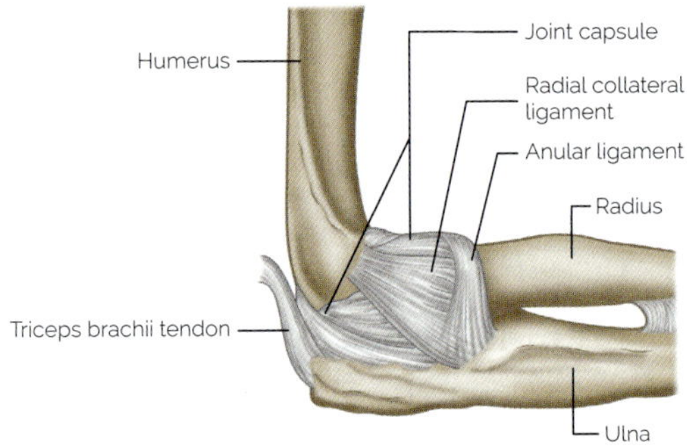

Figure II.2: Right elbow, lateral view.

CHAPTER 8

Medial and Lateral Epicondylalgia

At the distal end of the humerus there are two ridges known as the *medial* and *lateral epicondyles* (figure 8.1). Muscles of wrist flexion attach to the medial epicondyle (figure 8.2), and muscles of wrist extension attach to the lateral epicondyle (figure 8.3). As you may know, these muscles are also weak flexors and extensors of the elbow, respectively.

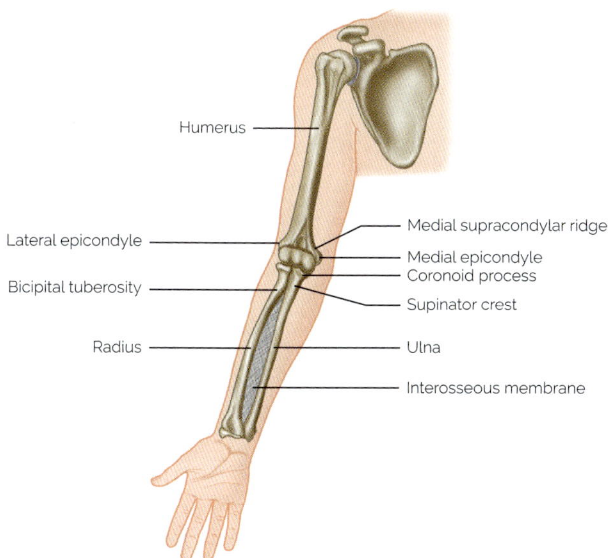

Figure 8.1: The medial and lateral epicondyles of the humerus.

It is from these anatomical regions that we get the terms *medial* and *lateral epicondylalgia*, commonly known as golfer's elbow and tennis elbow. The tests in this chapter will help you to identify these conditions in your clients. As their names suggest, the Golfer's Elbow Provocation Test and the Golfer's Elbow Test will help you to identify medial epicondylalgia, and Cozen's Test, Mill's Test and Maudsley's Test will help you to identify lateral epicondylalgia (tennis elbow). Polk's Test is a differentiation test designed to help you differentiate between medial and lateral epicondylalgia.

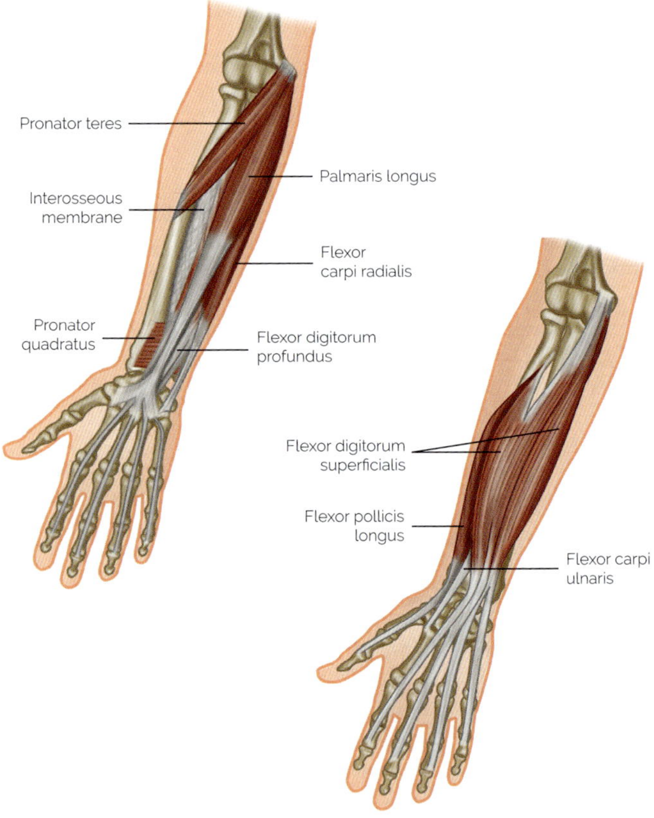

Figure 8.2: Muscles attaching to the medial epicondyle.

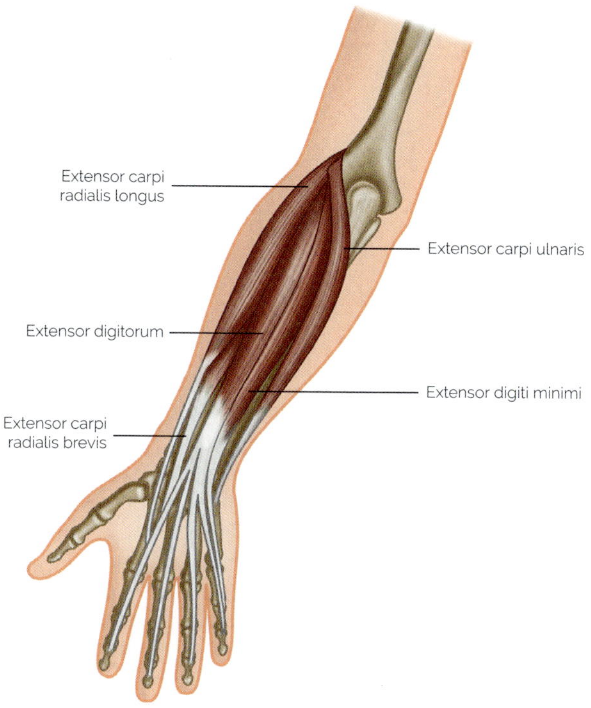

Figure 8.3: Muscles attaching to the lateral epicondyle.

Golfer's Elbow Provocation Test

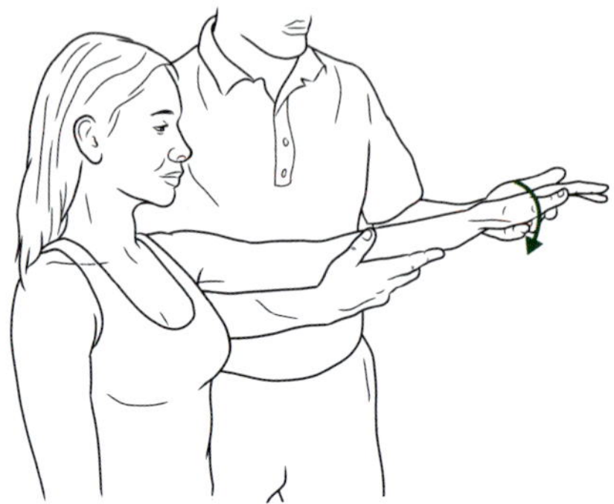

Figure 8.4: Golfer's Elbow Provocation Test, with an arrow indicating attempted wrist flexion.

Purpose: This tests for medial epicondylalgia.

Type of Test: This is a pain provocation test using isometric muscle contraction of the wrist and finger flexors.

Procedure: Begin with your client seated with their elbow extended and the forearm and wrist in pronation. Ask them to flex their wrist and fingers against resistance provided by you (figure 8.4).

Findings: The test is positive if there is pain at the medial epicondyle.

Tip: There are various ways to perform this test. Alternatives are for the examiner to form a fist and place this beneath the client's palm on the side being tested. Then, for the client to flex the fingers and wrist. Having a ball-shaped fist to grip and flex against can make it easier for some clients to perform the maneuver.

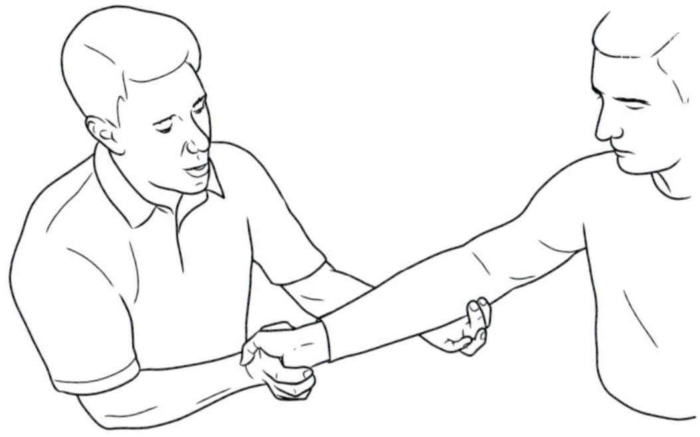

Figure 8.5: Golfer's Elbow Test.

Purpose: This is a test for medial epicondylalgia.

Type of Test: This is a passive pain-provocation test.

Procedure: Whilst palpating the medial epicondyle, passively supinate your client's forearm and then extend the elbow and wrist (figure 8.5).

Findings: The test is positive if there is pain at the medial epicondyle.

Tip: Amin, Kumar, and Schickendantz (2015) and Konarski et al. (2022) provide a useful description of medial epicondylalgia and other conditions affecting the elbow.

Cozen's Test

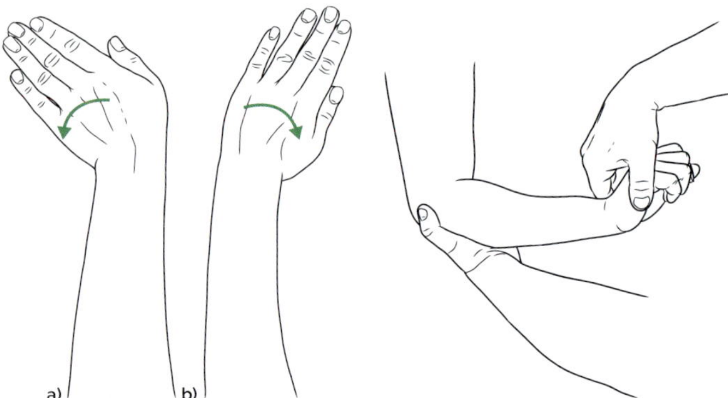

Figure 8.6: Ulnar (a) and radial (b) deviation of the wrist, with arrows indicating the direction of movement.

Figure 8.7: Cozen's Test, showing palpation of the lateral epicondyle whilst the client attempts isometric pronation, radial deviation, and extension of the wrist.

Purpose: This is a test for lateral epicondylalgia.

Type of Test: This is a pain provocation test using isometric contraction of the wrist extensors.

Procedure: Prior to this test it is useful to review ulnar (figure 8.6a) and radial (figure 8.6b) deviation. Palpate the lateral epicondyle of your client's symptomatic arm. Ask them to make a fist, pronate the forearm, and then radially deviate and extend the wrist against resistance provided by you (figure 8.7).

Findings: The test is positive if it provokes pain at the lateral epicondyle. In cases of severe lateral epicondylitis, pain will be elicited either on trying to maintain wrist extension or on resisted wrist extension.

Tip: Demonstrating radial deviation to your client prior to the test can be helpful. An alternative method is to ask your client to hold the position of wrist extension and radial deviation, and then for you to apply counterpressure (as if to move the wrist into flexion and ulnar deviation).

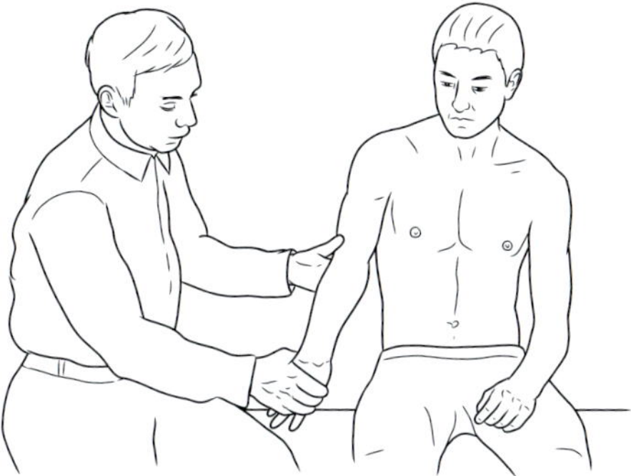

Figure 8.8: Mill's Test, showing passive pronation of the forearm, wrist flexion, and elbow extension, whilst the lateral epicondyle is palpated.

Purpose: This is a test for lateral epicondylalgia and stresses the radial nerve.

Type of Test: This is a passive pain-provocation test.

Procedure: The test is performed most easily with your client standing. Palpate the lateral epicondyle with one hand, then, using your other hand, passively pronate your client's forearm, fully flex the wrist, and extend the elbow (figure 8.8).

Findings: The test is positive if there is pain over the lateral epicondyle, but does not differentiate between lateral epicondylitis and radial nerve pathology.

Tip: As the forearm is pronated there is a tendency for the client to actively rotate their arm internally, but if the examiner retains their thumb on the lateral epicondyle, the results will be the same.

Maudsley's Test

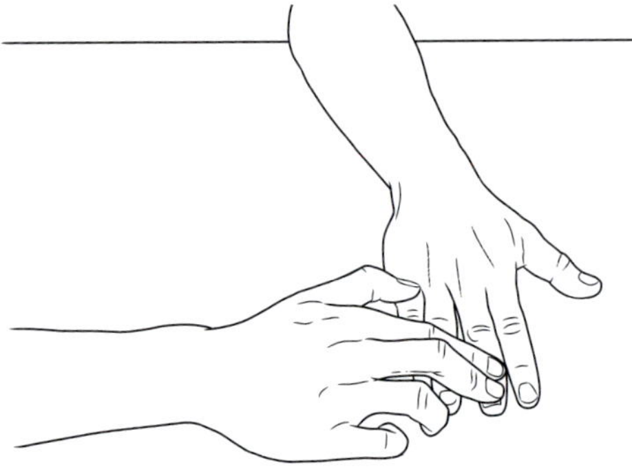

Figure 8.9: Maudsley's Test, involving attempted extension of the middle finger against resistance provided by the clinician.

Purpose: Described by Roles and Maudsley (1972), this tests for lateral epicondylalgia. Fairbank and Corlett (2002) provide an interesting view of the role of the extensor digitorum communis muscle in lateral epicondylalgia, with specific reference to the Maudsley test.

Type of Test: This is an active pain-provocation test involving isometric contraction of the extensor muscle of the middle finger.

Procedure: Begin with your client sitting, their hand palm down on a table, and the elbow extended. Ask them to extend their middle finger against resistance provided by you (figure 8.9).

Findings: The test is positive if there is pain at the lateral epicondyle.

Tip: Minimal resistance is required by the examiner, and therefore it is best to apply pressure to the dorsum of the tip of your client's middle finger using only your own finger.

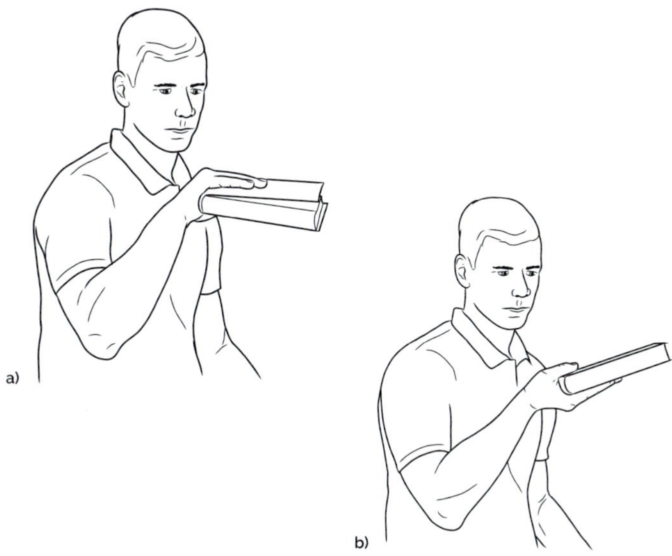

Figure 8.10: Polk's Test: (a) position for lateral epicondylalgia; (b) position for medial epicondylalgia.

Purpose: Described by Polkinghorn (2002), this test is designed to differentiate between lateral and medial epicondylalgia.

Type of Test: This is an active pain-provocation test involving concentric contraction of the muscles affected by lateral and medial epicondylalgia. It can be thought of as a motion stress test.

Procedure: Begin with your client seated. The test is first performed by lifting a heavy book with the forearm pronated (figure 8.10a), then lifting the same book with the forearm supinated (figure 8.10b).

Findings: The test is positive for lateral epicondylalgia if pain is felt at the lateral epicondyle when lifting the book with the forearm pronated, and positive for medial epicondylalgia if pain is felt in the medial epicondyle when lifting the book with the forearm supinated.

Tip: Any item weighing 5 lbs (2.3 kg) could be used instead of a book, provided the method of lifting remains the same.

CHAPTER 9

Stability Tests

As you learned from the introduction to this part of the book, the elbow comprises three joints, two of which are shown here. The hinge joint is formed by the distal end of the humerus and the proximal end of the ulna (figure 9.1a), and the pivot joint is formed by the proximal ends of the radius and ulna (figure 9.1b). This pivot joint is known as the *proximal radioulnar joint*, as there is another joint between the radius and ulna at the wrist, the *distal radioulnar joint*. The Valgus Stress Test, Varus Stress Test, and Moving Valgus Stress Test within this chapter will help you to identify laxity in these joints, and in the strong ligaments that protect them (figure 9.2).

Posterolateral instability of the elbow is characterized by subluxation or dislocation of the radial head relative to the capitellum, plus posterior displacement of the ulna relative to the trochlea.

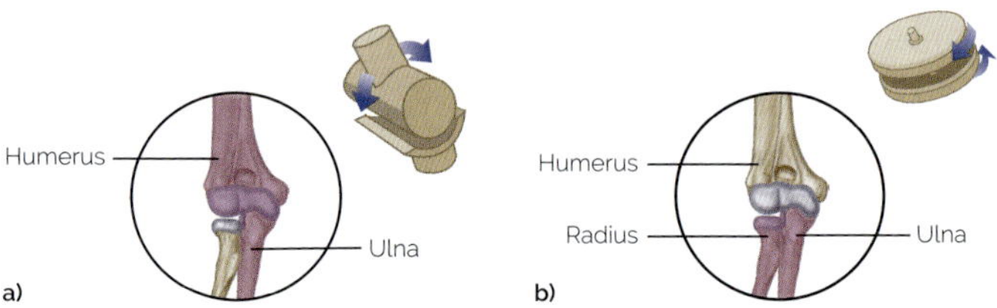

Figure 9.1: (a) Hinge joint of the elbow formed by the distal end of the humerus and the proximal end of the ulna; (b) pivot joint of the elbow formed by the proximal ends of the radius and ulna.

The Posterolateral Rotatory-Instability Test and the Chair Push-Up Test will specifically help you to identify whether there is loss of stability in the proximal superior radioulnar joint (figure 9.3).

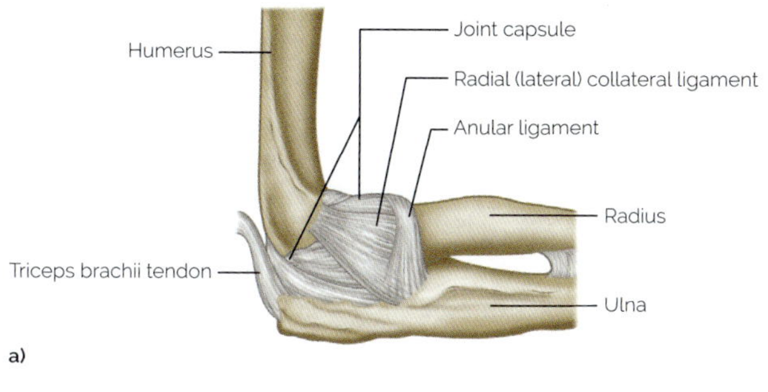

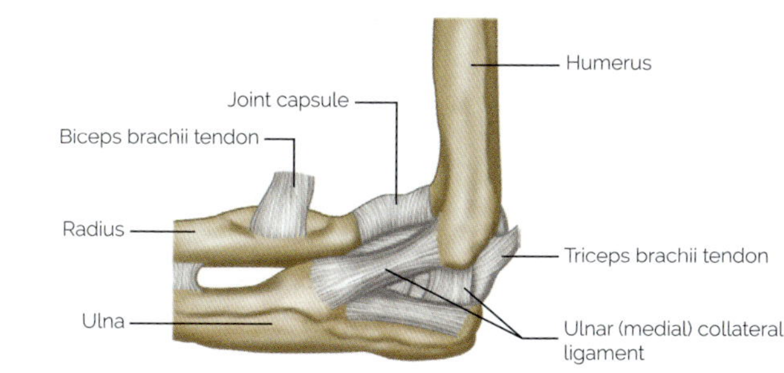

Figure 9.2: Ligaments of the right elbow: (a) lateral view; (b) medial view.

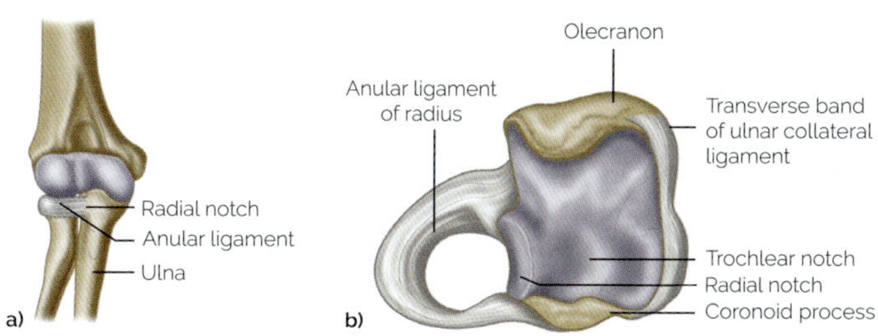

Figure 9.3: The anular ligament of the proximal superior radioulnar joint of the left elbow: (a) anterior view; (b) superior view.

Valgus Stress Test

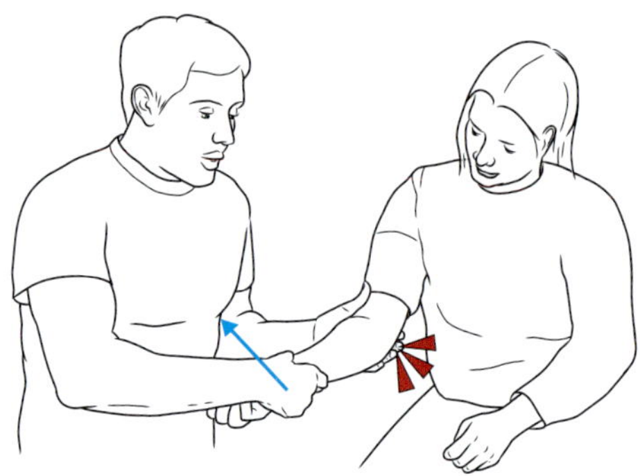

Figure 9.4: Valgus Stress Test, with arrow showing direction of clinician's pressure.

Purpose: This is a test for the integrity of the medial collateral ligament of the elbow (figure 9.2b).

Type of Test: This is a passive joint movement test.

Procedure: The test is performed with the arm in external rotation, the forearm supinated, and the elbow flexed to approximately 20°. Grasp and stabilize your client's arm with one hand, then abduct the forearm with respect to the humerus (figure 9.4). This stresses the medial collateral ligament.

Findings: The test is positive if there is localized pain or increased movement in the joint.

Tip: A good way to envisage the starting point for the arm when performing this test is as when a person is standing with the upper limbs in the anatomical position.

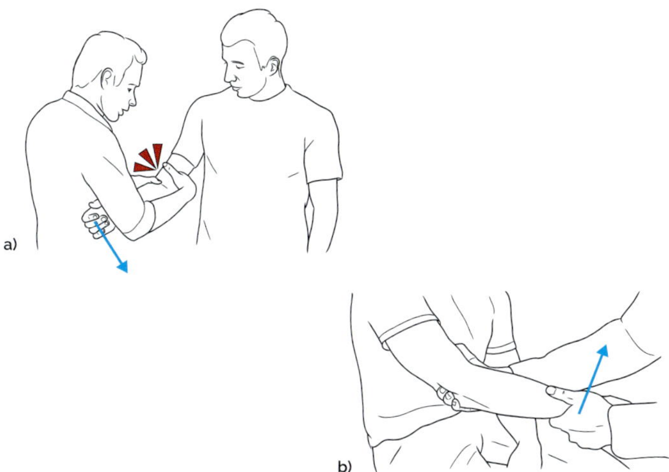

Figure 9.5: Alternative clinician handholds for the Varus Stress Test, with arrows showing the direction of passive force applied with the forearm in supination (a) or pronation (b).

Purpose: This tests for the integrity of the lateral collateral ligament of the elbow (figure 9.2a).

Type of Test: This is a passive joint movement test.

Procedure: The test may be performed in a variety of ways. One way is for you to fix the client's forearm as shown in figure 9.5a, with their elbow flexed to approximately 20°–30°. Next, grasp and stabilize the arm in one hand and the forearm in the other, and apply an opposing force, thus stressing the lateral collateral ligament. An alternative method is with the client's arm adducted across the body and the forearm pronated; you then apply a varus force by moving your client's forearm with respect to the humerus (figure 9.5b).

Findings: The test is positive if there is localized pain or increased movement in the joint.

Tip: Although the clinician has better leverage on the forearm when holding the wrist, the key with this test is to ensure that the ligament is tensioned. Therefore, it may be necessary to experiment with different handholds to achieve this, based on the body size of the client with respect to the examiner.

Moving Valgus Stress Test

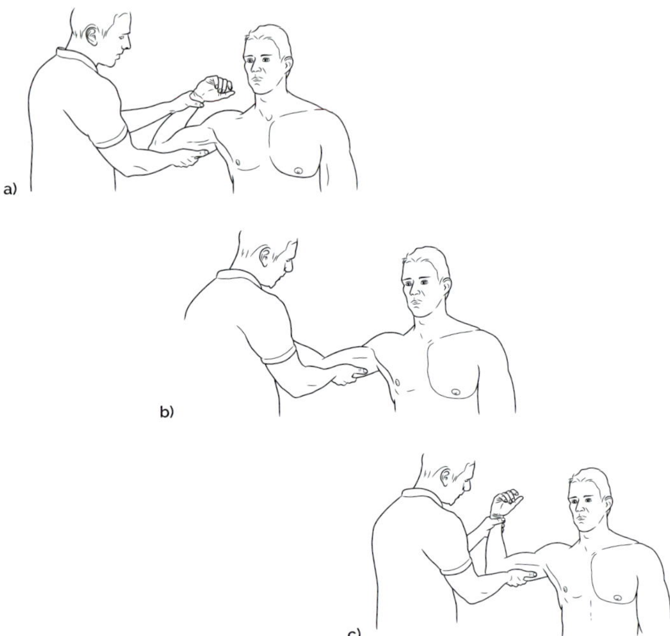

Figure 9.6: Moving Valgus Stress Test: (a) start position; (b) maximal external rotation of the shoulder with a valgus torque force applied followed by quick elbow extension to 30°; (c) a positive test is indicated by pain in the range of 70°–120° of elbow flexion.

Purpose: This tests for instability in the medial collateral ligament of the elbow (figure 9.2b).

Type of Test: This is a passive pain-provocation test.

Procedure: The test begins with your client standing, with their arm abducted to 90° and the elbow fully flexed (figure 9.6a). The shoulder is maximally externally rotated. Apply a valgus torque to the elbow then quickly extend the elbow to approximately 30° (figure 9.6b).

Findings: The test is positive if there is sudden elbow pain that is familiar to the client and maximal between 70° and 120° of elbow flexion (figure 9.6c).

Tip: It is important to maintain the valgus torque throughout the maneuver.

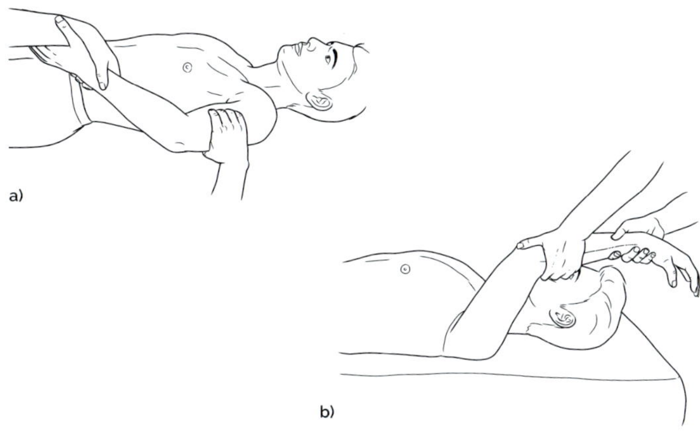

Figure 9.7: Posterolateral Rotatory-Instability Test of the Elbow: (a) with the client supine; (b) with the arm above the head.

Purpose: Described by O'Driscoll, Bell, and Morrey (1991), this tests for posterolateral rotatory-instability of the elbow plus integrity of the lateral collateral ligament of the elbow (figure 9.2a).

Type of Test: This is a passive joint movement test.

Procedure: O'Driscoll et al. describe two test positions: With your client either in the supine position (figure 9.7a) or with their arm above their head (figure 9.7b), internally rotate the shoulder and supinate the forearm. Begin with the elbow fully extended, then, maintaining the forearm in supination, apply axial pressure through the forearm toward the elbow, and apply a valgus force to the elbow.

Findings: The test is positive if there is pain or apprehension.

Chair Push-Up Test

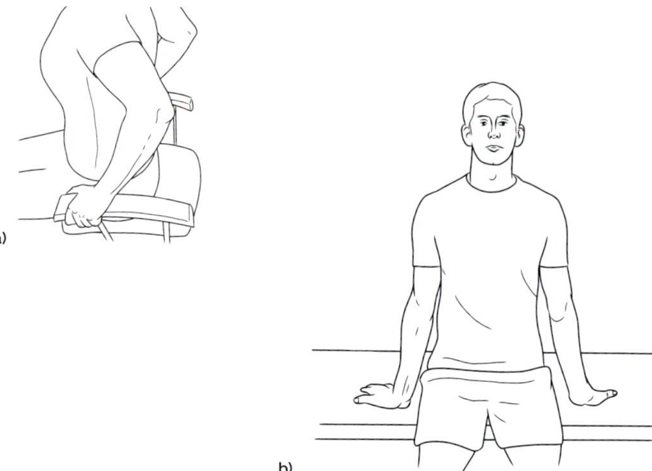

Figure 9.8: Chair Push-Up Test: (a) with the forearm in part supination; (b) with the forearm in full supination.

Purpose: This tests for posterolateral rotatory instability and integrity of the lateral collateral ligament of the elbow (figure 9.2a).

Type of Test: This is a function test involving axial pressure through the forearm and into the elbow joint.

Procedure: Begin with your client sitting on a chair with arms, their hands resting on the arms of the chair (figure 9.8a) or a treatment plinth (figure 9.8b). In this position the elbows are flexed. Ask your client to place weight through their arms as if attempting to stand up from their sitting position.

Findings: The test is positive if there is apprehension, pain, locking, or clicking.

Tip: The test is best performed in a variety of start positions ranging from part supination (figure 9.8a) to full supination (figure 9.8b) and pronation of the wrist, as instability can be positional.

CHAPTER 10

Nerve Compression Tests

The ulnar (figure 10.1) and radial (figure 10.2) nerves may be compressed at the elbow. Compression can affect both the motor and sensory functions of these nerves. Compression of the ulnar nerve at the elbow is known as *cubital tunnel syndrome*.

This chapter contains four tests that will help you to assess for entrapment of these nerves. Three of the tests are for assessment of the ulnar nerve: the Ulnar Nerve Flexion Test, the Pressure Provocation Test, and Tinel's Test (or Hoffman-Tinel Sign).
The Supinator Compression Test is included for assessment of the radial nerve.

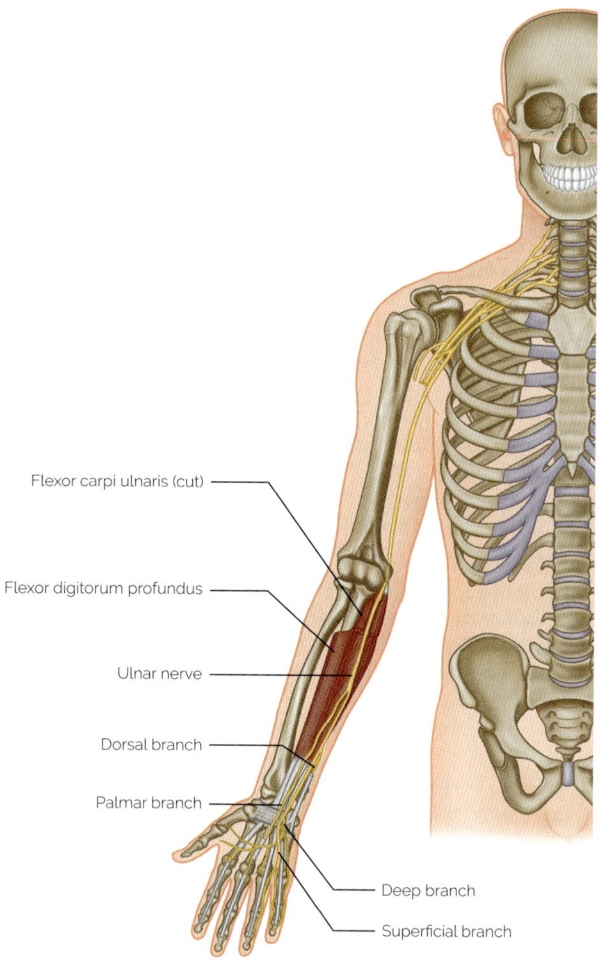

Figure 10.1: Motor pathway of the ulnar nerve.

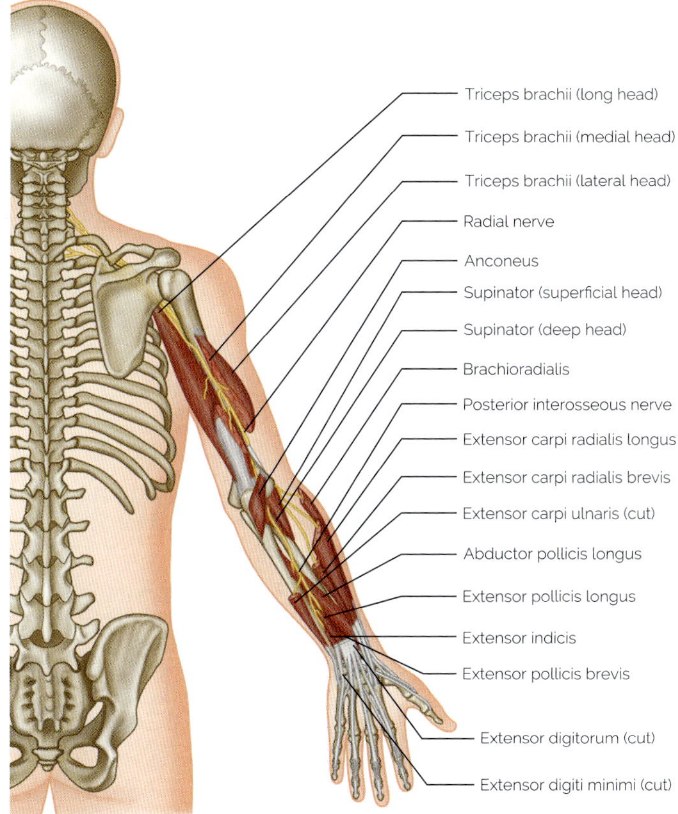

Figure 10.2: Motor pathway of the radial nerve.

Ulnar Nerve Flexion Test

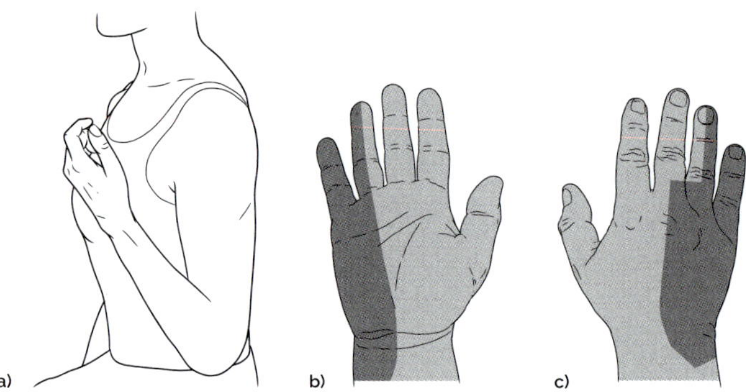

Figure 10.3: Position for the Ulnar Nerve Flexion Test (a), which is positive when there is pain or numbness in the sensory distribution of the palmar side (b) and dorsum (c) of the hand.

Purpose: This tests for cubital tunnel syndrome (compression of the ulnar nerve at the elbow).

Type of Test: This is an active nerve compression test.

Procedure: Ask your client to supinate their forearm and then fully flex the elbow whilst keeping the wrist in a neutral position (figure 10.3a). The client maintains this position for 60 seconds.

Findings: The test is positive if it elicits pain, paresthesia, or numbness in the sensory distribution of the ulnar nerve on the palmar side (figure 10.3b) and dorsum (figure 10.3c) of the hand.

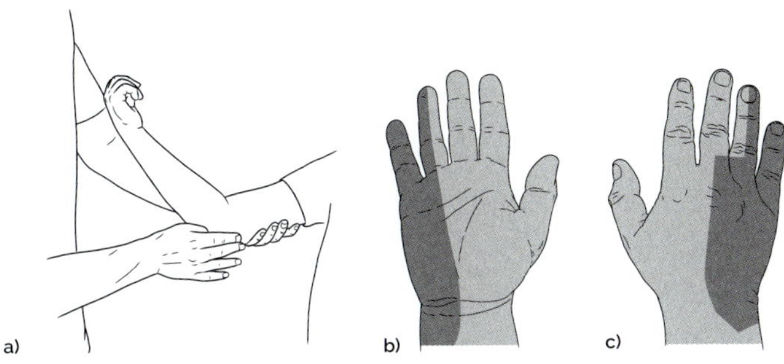

Figure 10.4: Point of palpation for the Pressure Provocation Test (a); a positive test is indicated by pain, paresthesia, or numbness in the sensory distribution of the ulnar nerve on the palmar side (b) and dorsum (c) of the hand.

Purpose: This tests for cubital tunnel syndrome (compression of the ulnar nerve at the elbow).

Type of Test: This is a passive symptom-provocation test involving compression of the ulnar nerve.

Procedure: With your client seated, passively flex their elbow to approximately 20°, supinate the forearm, and locate the ulnar nerve. This lies in the groove between the posterior aspect of the medial epicondyle of the humerus and the olecranon. It can be palpated as a cord-like structure proximal to the cubital tunnel. Using your index finger, apply pressure to the nerve at this spot for 60 seconds (figure 10.4a).

Findings: The test is positive if it elicits pain, paresthesia, or numbness in the sensory distribution of the ulnar nerve on the palmar side (figure 10.4b) and dorsum (figure 10.4c) of the hand.

Tinel's Test or Hoffman-Tinel Sign

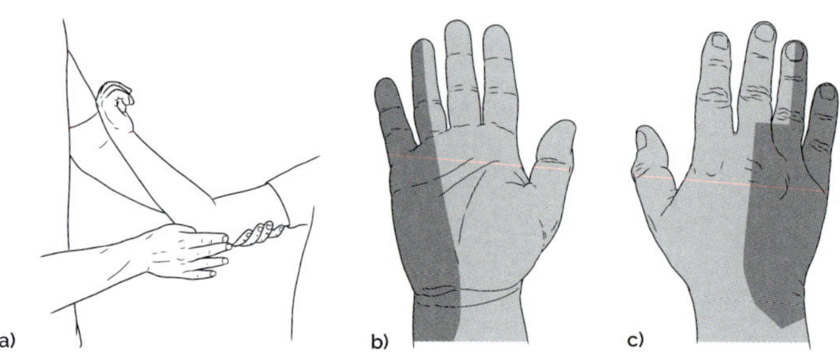

Figure 10.5: Position for the Tinel's Test of the elbow (a); a positive test is indicated by paresthesia or numbness in the sensory distribution of the ulnar nerve on the palmar side (b) and dorsum (c) of the hand.

Purpose: Described in 2015 by both Jules Tinel (translated as Tinel 1971) and Paul Hoffman, this tests for cubital tunnel syndrome (compression of the ulnar nerve at the elbow).

Type of Test: This is a passive symptom-provocation test involving compression of the ulnar nerve.

Procedure: With your client sitting or standing, locate the ulnar nerve at the elbow. This lies in the groove between the posterior aspect of the medial epicondyle of the humerus and the olecranon. It can be palpated as a cord-like structure proximal to the cubital tunnel. Tinel indicated that when the nerve was compressed it elicits symptoms. Hoffman suggested applying percussion using a finger (figure 10.5a), reflex hammer, or thumb pressure.

Findings: The test is positive if there is paresthesia in the sensory distribution of the ulnar nerve on the palmar side (figure 10.5b) and dorsum (figure 10.5c) of the hand.

Tip: Siqueira and Martins (2023) provide a comprehensive overview of the historical background and clinical significance of the Hoffman-Tinel Sign.

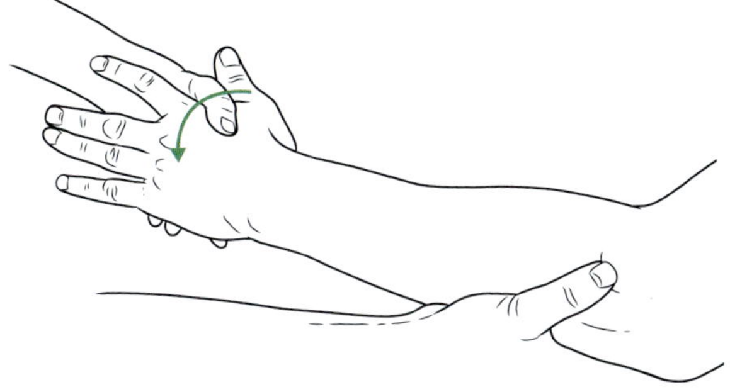

Figure 10.6: Supinator Compression Test, with an arrow showing attempted supination of the forearm by the client.

Purpose: This tests for entrapment of the deep branch of the radial nerve at the arcade of Frohse, also known as the supinator arch. The arch is formed by two bands of the supinator muscle.

Type of Test: It involves isometric supination with simultaneous passive palpation of the supinator muscle.

Procedure: Locate the supinator muscle. Whilst applying gentle pressure to this point, ask your client to supinate their forearm against resistance.

Findings: The test is positive if there is soreness at the site of palpation and/or temporary weakness in active supination.

CHAPTER 11

Soft Tissue Tests

A fold in the synovial tissue of the elbow is known as a *synovial plica* (figure 11.1). Although uncommon, synovial plica syndrome causes pain in the lateral aspect of the elbow and when the elbow is in full extension. It has been included here because the symptoms of this condition can mimic those of lateral epicondylalgia, and it is therefore useful to be able to differentiate between the two.

The Elbow Plica Entrapment Test (Flexion-Pronation) is used to assess lateral plica, whilst the Elbow Plica Entrapment Test (Extension-Supination) is used for assessment of posterior plica. Also included in this chapter is the Elbow Hook Test to assess rupture of the distal tendon of the biceps brachii muscle, as this too is an important soft tissue structure.

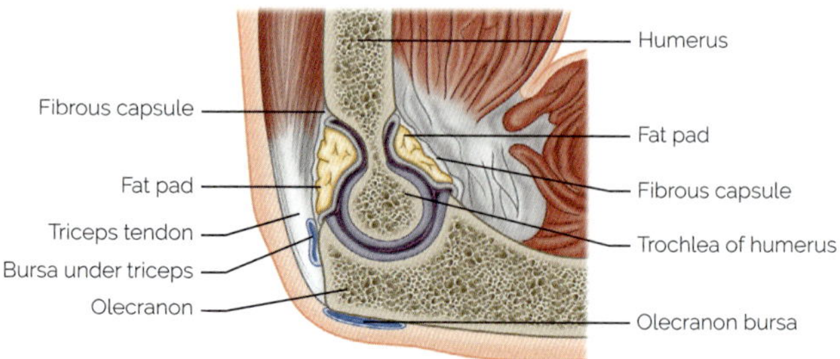

Figure 11.1: Mid-sagittal view of the elbow of the right arm, showing the synovium, which may become symptomatic when trapped.

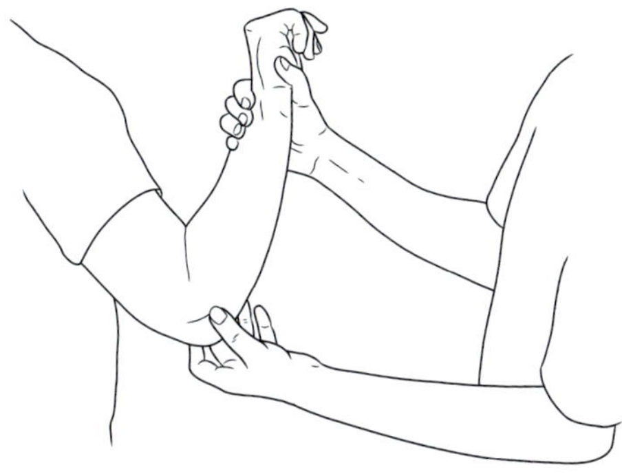

Figure 11.2: Elbow Plica Entrapment (Flexion-Pronation) Test.

Purpose: Described by Antuna and O'Driscoll (2001), this tests for entrapment of the lateral plica of the elbow.

Type of Test: This is a passive test combining palpation with movement.

Procedure: With your client's elbow extended and the forearm pronated, apply gentle pressure to the lateral side of the radiohumeral joint using your thumb. Maintaining pressure, gently flex the elbow (figure 11.2).

Findings: The test is positive if there is a palpable snap beneath your thumb at approximately 90° of elbow flexion. This may be accompanied by pain at the anterolateral or posterolateral aspect of the elbow.

Elbow Plica Entrapment (Extension-Supination) Test

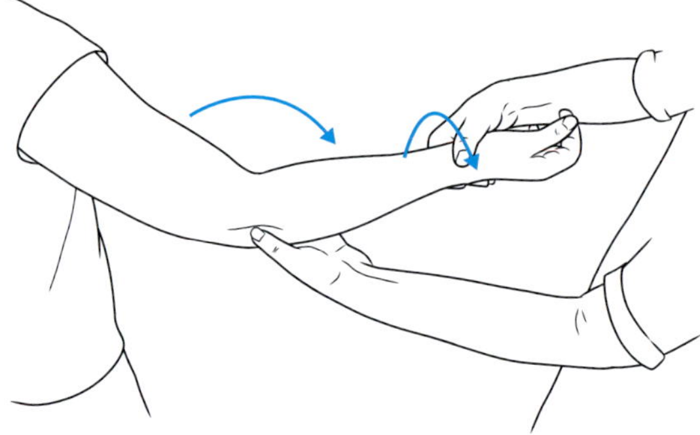

Figure 11.3: Elbow Plica Entrapment (Extension-Supination) Test.

Purpose: This tests for entrapment of the posterior plica of the elbow.

Type of Test: This is a passive test combining palpation with movement.

Procedure: With your client's elbow flexed and the forearm supinated, place your thumb on the arthroscopic soft spot of the elbow. Maintaining pressure, extend the elbow (figure 11.3).

Findings: The test is positive if at almost full extension there is a palpable snap beneath the examiner's thumb.

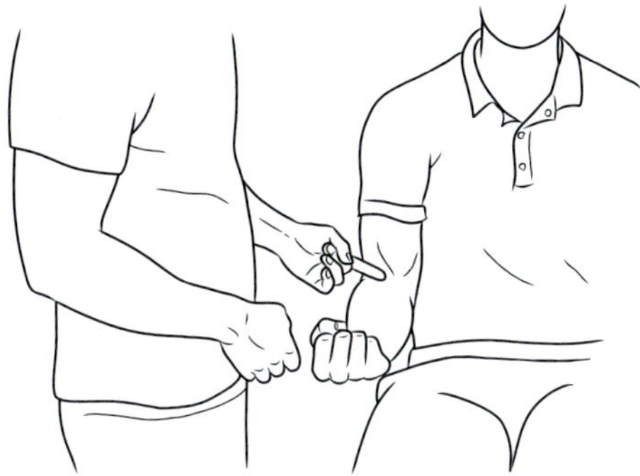

Figure 11.4: Elbow Hook Test.

Purpose: Described by O'Driscoll, Goncalves, and Dietz (2007), this tests for rupture of the distal tendon of biceps brachii.

Type of Test: This is a passive test.

Procedure: Ask your client to actively flex their elbow to 90° and fully supinate their forearm. Attempt to hook your index finger beneath the distal tendon of biceps brachii from the lateral side of the elbow (figure 11.4). An intact tendon feels like a cord.

Findings: The test is positive if there is no tendon to "hook."

PART III

THE WRIST AND HAND

The wrist comprises the distal ends of the radius and ulna bones plus the carpal bones (figure III.1). The eight carpal bones are scaphoid, lunate, triquetrum, trapezium, trapezoid, capitate, hamate, and pisiform.

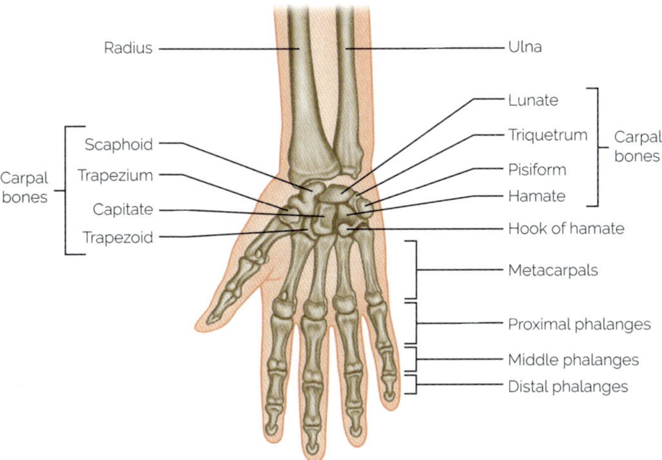

Figure III.1: Anterior view of the bones of the right wrist and hand.

There are two joints known as *compound joints*, and these are the radiocarpal joint and midcarpal joint. Together these are known as the wrist complex. You can see from figure III.2 that the radiocarpal joint is formed by the articulation of the radius with the proximal row of carpal bones—the scaphoid, lunate, and triquetrum. Notice that there is an articular disc at the head of the ulna. This too forms part of the radiocarpal joint.

You can also see from figure III.2 that the three scaphoid bones of the radiocarpal joint—the scaphoid, lunate, and triquetrum—also articulate with the trapezium, the trapezoid, the capitate, and the hamate bones to form the midcarpal joint.

This part includes 15 tests for the wrist and hand plus one test for the fingers. Special tests are used primarily to assess the integrity of ligaments (chapter 12), but also included are three important carpal tunnel tests (chapter 13) and two tests for the thumb (chapter 14).

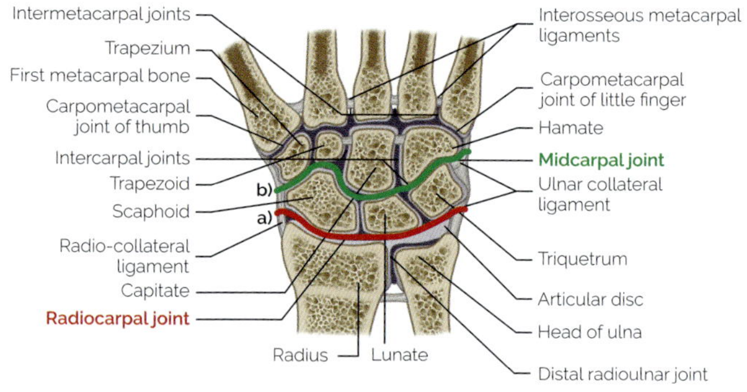

Figure III.2: The radiocarpal joint (a) and the midcarpal joint (b).

CHAPTER 12

Wrist Ligament Tests

There are multiple ligaments supporting the bones of the wrist and hand, with a complex arrangement and function. A simple way to think about these is according to whether they are intrinsic or extrinsic. Intrinsic ligaments are those that connect the bones of the carpals and are therefore sometimes known as *intercarpal ligaments* or even *interosseous ligaments*. They lie within the synovial lining of the wrist. Extrinsic ligaments lie outside of the synovial lining of the wrist and connect the carpals to the radius or ulna proximally, or to the metacarpals distally. A selection of 10 commonly used special tests has been included in this chapter. The radial collateral ligament and the ulnar collateral ligament (figure 12.1) are examples of extrinsic

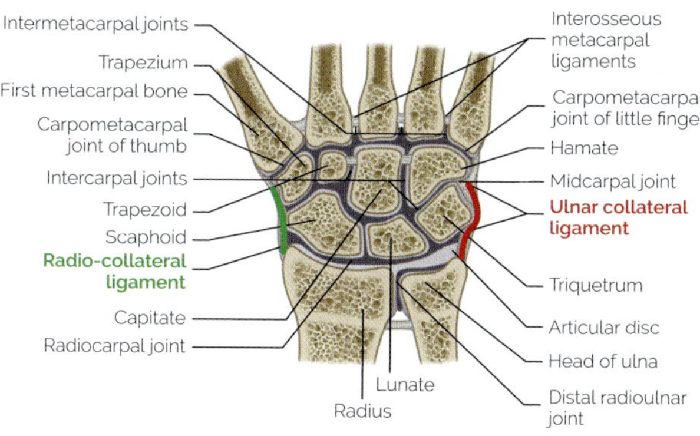

Figure 12.1: Radial collateral and ulnar collateral ligaments of the wrist.

ligaments, and their tests are perhaps the easiest to perform. The function of the radial collateral ligament is to limit ulnar deviation, whilst the function of the ulnar collateral ligament is to limit radial deviation. The Radial Collateral Ligament Stress Test and the Ulnar Collateral Ligament Stress Test included in this chapter will help you to assess these ligaments by utilizing the movements of ulnar and radial deviation.

The arrangement of ligaments in the wrist has been found to vary widely between individuals. This may account for why different clinicians have developed tests for the same ligament that involve subtle variations. A good example of this is in the variety of tests for the lunotriquetral joint, of which four are provided here. Also included is the Piano Key Test (used to assess the distal radioulnar joint), the Watson Test (which tests the scapholunate ligament), and the Dorsal Capitate Displacement Apprehension Test (to help you to determine whether the capitate bone is displaced). The Supination Lift Test has also been included, as this tests for the triangular fibrocartilage complex (TFCC). The TFCC comprises a fibrocartilage disc as well as radioulnar and ulnocarpal ligaments.

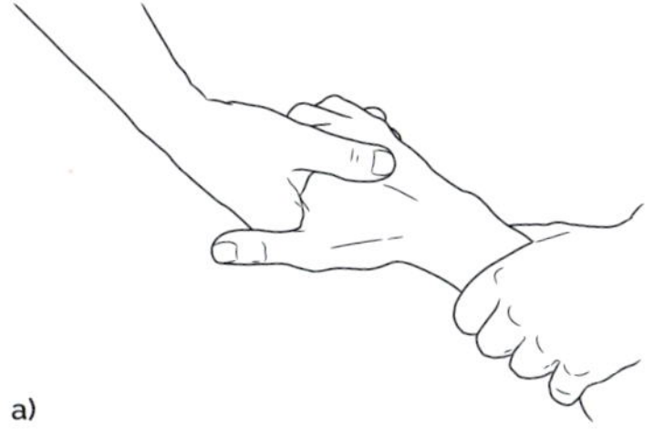

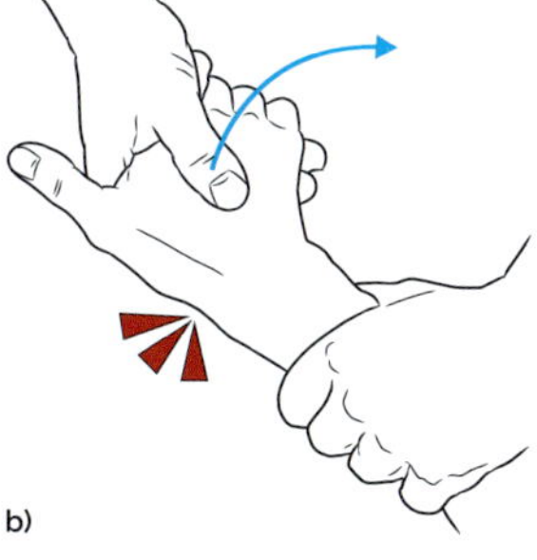

Figure 12.2: Radial Collateral Ligament Stress Test: (a) start position; (b) with the wrist in ulnar deviation.

Purpose: This tests for integrity of the radial collateral ligament.

Type of Test: This is a passive joint movement test that stresses the radial collateral ligament.

Procedure: The clinician grasps the client's forearm superior to the wrist, and with their other hand, holds the hand (figure 12.2a). The wrist is then moved into ulnar deviation (figure 12.2b), thus stressing the radial collateral ligament of the wrist.

Findings: The test is positive if there is pain on the radial aspect of the wrist and/or joint laxity.

Tip: It is important not to involve the client's fingers or thumb but to let these rest in their neutral positions.

Ulnar Collateral Ligament Stress Test

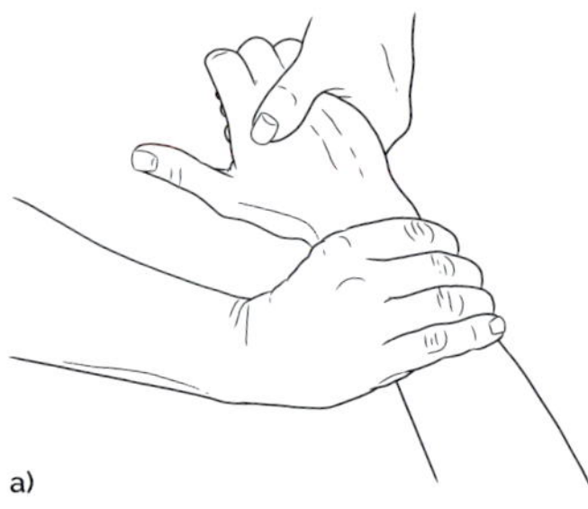

a)

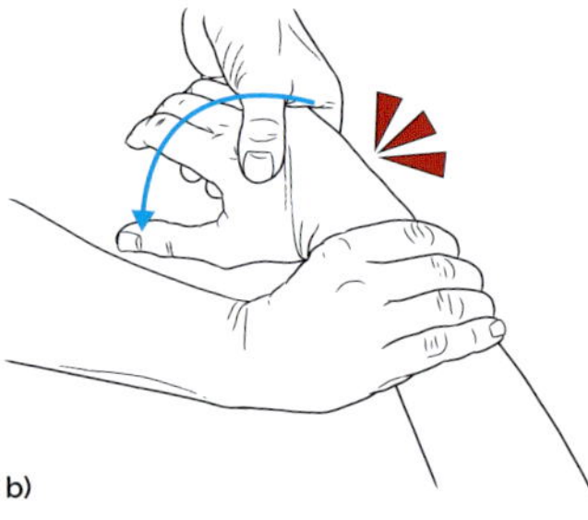

b)

Figure 12.3: Ulnar Collateral Ligament Stress Test: (a) start position; (b) with the wrist in radial deviation.

Purpose: This tests for integrity of the ulnar collateral ligament.

Type of Test: This is a passive joint movement test.

Procedure: The clinician grasps the client's forearm superior to the wrist, and with their other hand, holds the hand (figure 12.3a). The wrist is then moved into radial deviation (figure 12.3b), thus stressing the ulnar collateral ligament of the wrist.

Findings: The test is positive if there is pain on the ulnar aspect of the wrist and/or joint laxity.

Tip: It is important not to involve the client's fingers or thumb but to let these rest in their neutral positions.

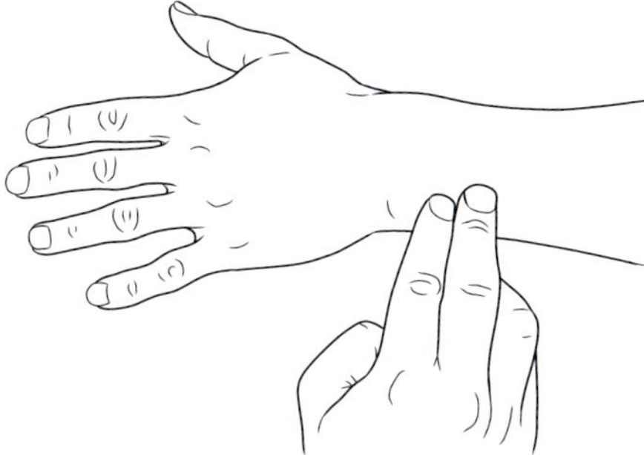

Figure 12.4: Piano Key Test.

Purpose: This tests for integrity of the distal radioulnar joint. For a helpful discussion of the anatomy and physical examination of ulnar-sided wrist pain, see Vezeridis et al. (2010).

Type of Test: This is a passive joint movement test.

Procedure: Ask your client to sit with their forearms in pronation. Use one or more fingers to gently press down on the head of the ulna as though you were depressing a piano key (figure 12.4). Repeat the test on the client's other wrist.

Findings: The test is positive if there is a difference in joint mobility between the left and right wrists and/or the test elicits pain. There should be minimal movement in an intact joint. Where the ulna springs back into place like a piano key, this is indicative of a positive test (Vezeridis et al. 2010).

Watson (Scaphoid Shift) Test

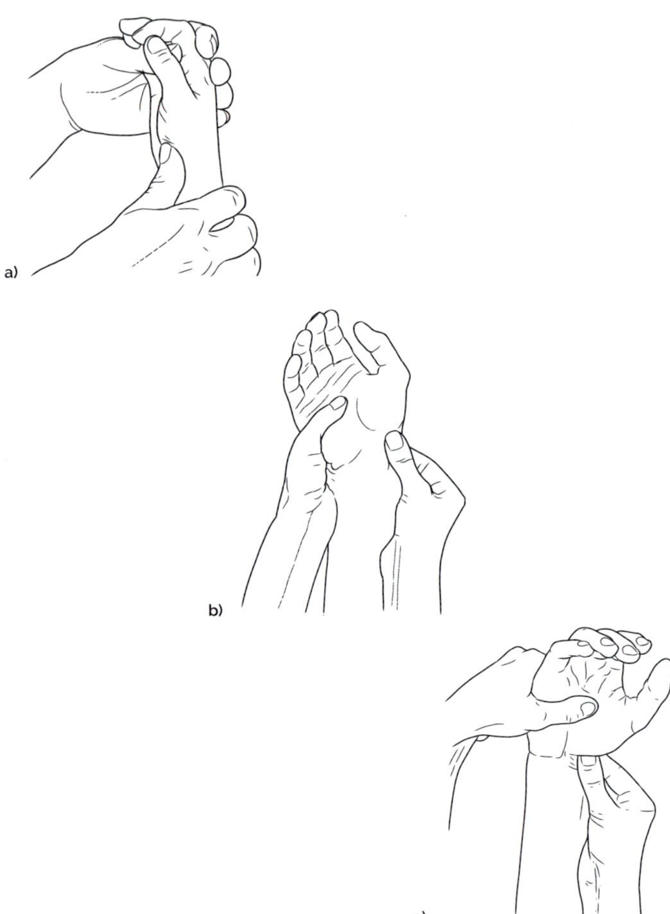

Figure 12.5: The Watson Scaphoid Shift Test: (a) beginning with the application of thumb pressure on the palmar prominence of the scaphoid whilst applying counterpressure with the fingers; (b) the wrist is moved into ulnar deviation with slight extension; (c) the wrist is then moved into radial deviation and slight flexion.

Purpose: Described by Watson, Ashmead, and Makhlouf (1988), this tests for integrity of the scapholunate ligament of the wrist.

Type of Test: This is a passive joint movement test.

Procedure: With the client's forearm slightly pronated and the wrist in ulnar deviation with slight extension, grasp the wrist on the radial side and apply thumb pressure on the palmar prominence of the scaphoid whilst applying counterpressure with the fingers (figure 12.5a). Maintaining pressure on the scaphoid, move the wrist into the start position of ulnar deviation with slight extension (figure 12.5b), and then to radial deviation and slight flexion (figure 12.5c). This thumb pressure creates a subluxation stress and may result in a scaphoid "shift."

Findings: Watson, Ashmead, and Makhlouf point out that the test is a provocative maneuver that does not yield a positive or negative result but rather a variety of findings, which may be interpreted depending on the skill of the clinician. However, if the scaphoid shifts during the maneuver and when the examiner removes their thumb pressure, the scaphoid returns to its resting position with a "thunk" sound, this is likely to be indicative of loss of integrity of the scapholunate ligament.

Tip: Watson, Ashmead, and Makhlouf suggest the following sitting position to perform the test: the client and examiner face each other seated at a table as if to perform arm wrestling, their elbows resting on the table. The examiner uses their right hand to assess the client's right wrist, and their left hand to examine the client's left wrist.

Lunotriquetral Shear Test

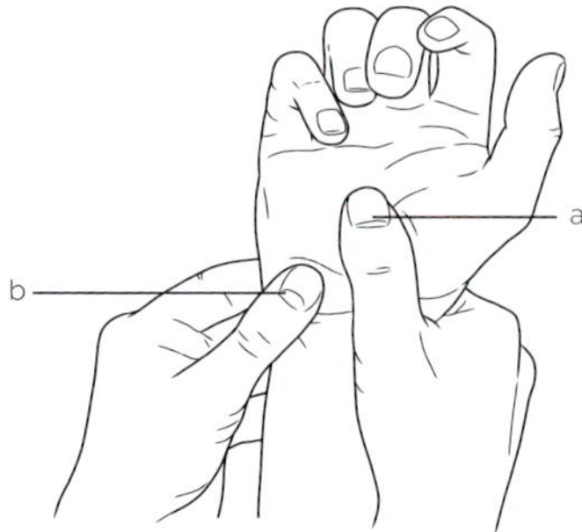

Figure 12.6: Lunotriquetral Shear Test, which involves holding the proximal row of carpals (a) and pressing the pisotriquetral joint (b).

Purpose: This tests for integrity of the lunotriquetral ligament.

Type of Test: This is a passive joint movement test.

Procedure: The client is seated with their elbow flexed in a neutral position. Hold the wrist by placing your thumb on the client's palm and your fingers supporting the proximal row of carpals on the dorsum (figure 12.6a). In this way the lunate is supported. Using your other hand, press the pisotriquetral joint (figure 12.6b) and apply a shearing force to the lunotriquetral (LT) joint.

Findings: The test is positive if there is laxity, crepitus, or pain.

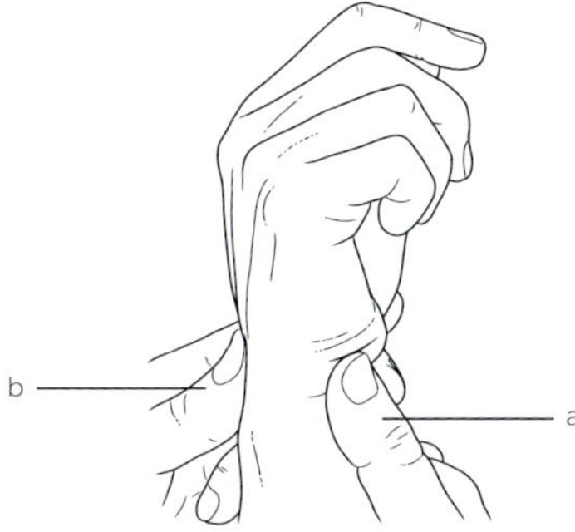

Figure 12.7: Kleinman's Lunotriquetral Shear Test: To assess the right LT joint the examiner places their right thumb over the palmar aspect of pisiform (a) and their left thumb over the dorsal aspect of lunate (b).

Purpose: Described by Kleinman (2015), this tests for instability of the LT joint.

Type of Test: This is a passive joint movement test.

Procedure: The client rests with their elbow on a table and the forearm in a neutral position, fingers pointing toward the ceiling. Use both of your hands to stabilize the hand-forearm during the test. To assess the right LT joint, place your right thumb over the palmar aspect of pisiform (figure 12.7a). Place your left thumb over the dorsal aspect of lunate (figure 12.7b). Apply pressure firmly to pisiform whilst your opposing thumb supports the dorsum of lunate. The maneuver shears the LT joint.

Findings: The test is positive if there is pain at the LT joint.

Tip: Kleinman advises to rule out pisotriquetral pathology before conducting the shear test.

Lunotriquetral Shear Test (Raegan)

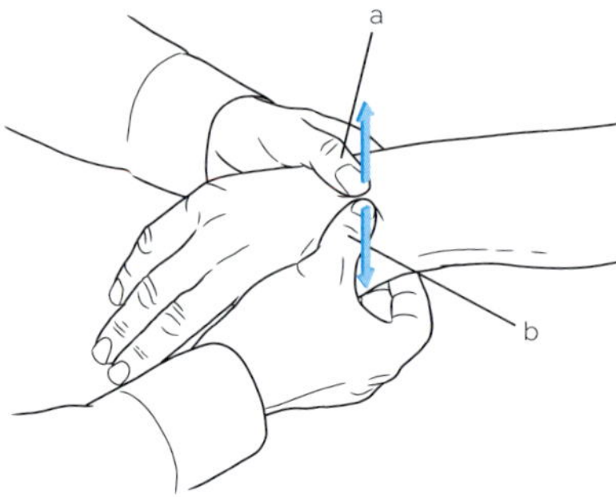

Figure 12.8: Raegan's Lunotriquetral Shear Test, which involves grasping the triquetrum bone (a) and moving the lunate bone (b) palmarly and dorsally.

Purpose: This tests for integrity of the lunotriquetral ligament.

Type of Test: This is a passive joint movement test.

Procedure: Using a pincer grip, grasp the triquetrum (figure 12.8a) between the thumb and forefinger of one hand, and similarly grasp the lunate (figure 12.8b) with the other. Lunate is then moved palmarly and dorsally.

Findings: The test is positive if there is laxity, crepitus, or pain.

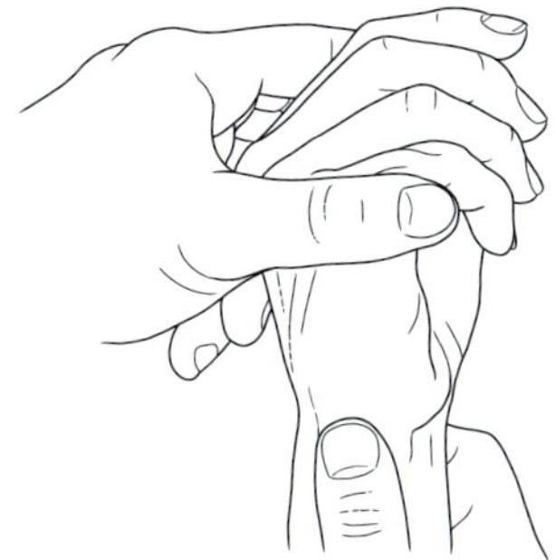

Figure 12.9: Linscheid's Lunotriquetral Shear Test involves compressing the triquetrum bone against the lunate bone.

Purpose: Described by Kleinman (2015), who attributes this to Linscheid, this is a crude test for integrity of the lunotriquetral ligament.

Type of Test: This is a passive joint compression test.

Procedure: With the client's forearm and wrist in a neutral position, use your thumb to apply pressure to the medial border of the triquetrum (figure 12.9), compressing it against the medial border of the lunate, the lunotriquetral ligament.

Findings: Pain at the site of pressure suggests damage to the LT joint.

Tip: Kleinman points out that false positives are common owing to the amount of force required to perform the test, which stresses the ulnocarpal ligaments, triangular fibrocartilage complex, and the extrinsic radiocarpal ligaments.

Dorsal Capitate Displacement Apprehension Test

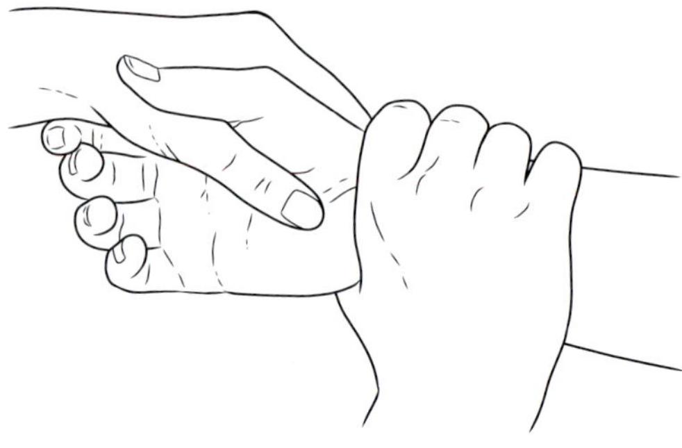

Figure 12.10: Dorsal Capitate Displacement Apprehension Test.

Purpose: This tests for the stability of the capitate bone.

Type of Test: This is a passive joint movement test.

Procedure: Hold your client's forearm at the wrist. Using your other hand, grasp their hand as shown in figure 12.10, to keep it in a neutral position. That is, with neither flexion nor extension and with neither radial nor ulnar deviation. Use your thumb in the position shown to push the capitate bone posteriorly, against counterpressure provided by your fingers of the same hand.

Findings: The test is positive if it elicits apprehension or pain, sometimes accompanied by a click.

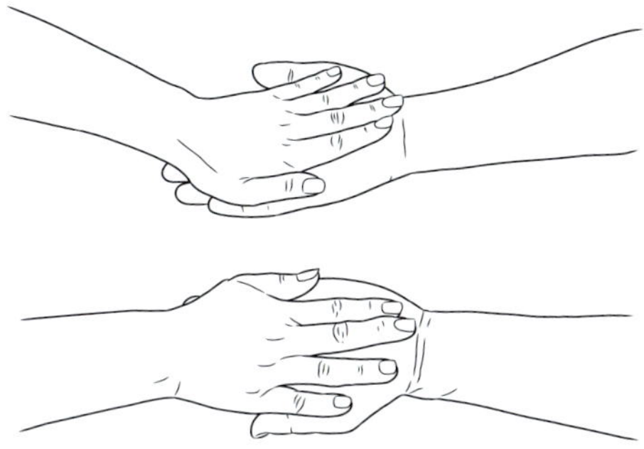

Figure 12.11: Supination Lift Test.

Purpose: This tests for integrity of the TFCC (figure 12.11).

Type of Test: This is an active test requiring isometric contraction of the elbow flexors.

Procedure: The client sits with their elbows flexed to 90° and forearms supinated. Place your hands over theirs, palm to palm. The client then attempts to flex their elbows, raising their hands against your counterpressure.

Findings: The test is positive if there is localized pain on the ulnar side of the wrist and difficulty performing the maneuver.

Tip: Tuhi (2023) provides a helpful overview of the diagnostic accuracy of tests for TFCC.

CHAPTER 13

Carpal Tunnel Tests

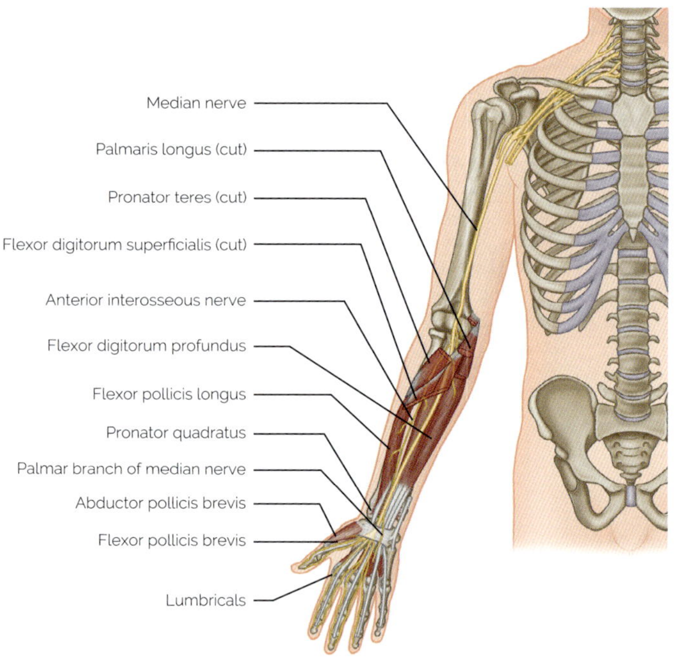

Figure 13.1: Motor pathway of the median nerve.

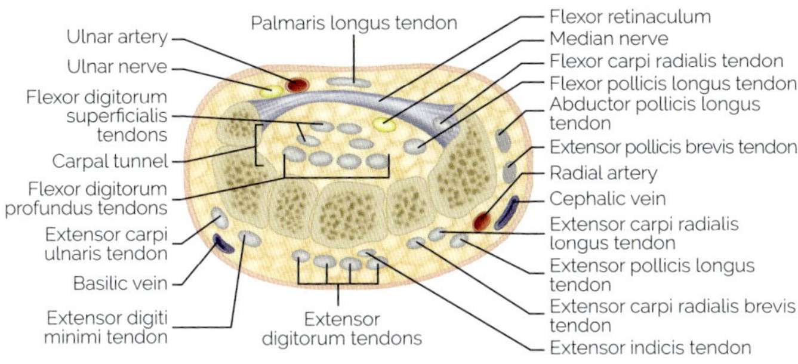

Figure 13.2: The carpal tunnel is a narrow passageway formed anteriorly at the wrist by the carpal bones and the flexor retinaculum, and serves as the entrance to the palm for several tendons and the median nerve. Here is a cross-section of the carpal tunnel, clearly showing the interrelationship between the muscles and associated structures. Note that the ulnar artery, ulnar nerve, and the tendon of the palmaris longus pass into the hand anterior to the flexor retinaculum, and so do not pass through the carpal tunnel.

Carpal tunnel syndrome involves compression of the median nerve (figure 13.1) in the carpal tunnel of the wrist (figure 13.2). This is a condition commonly encountered by musculoskeletal clinicians, and therefore three special tests for it have been included in this chapter. These are Tinel's Sign, Phalen's Test, and the Carpal Compression Test. When positive, these tests each elicit symptoms in the sensory function of the median nerve (figure 13.3).

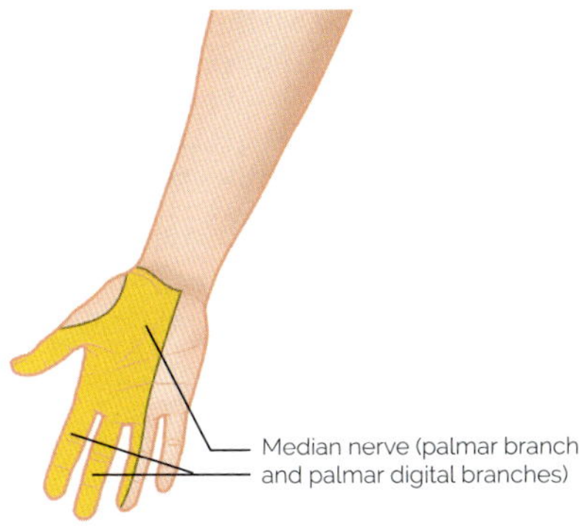

Figure 13.3: Sensory function of the median nerve.

Tinel's Sign Test

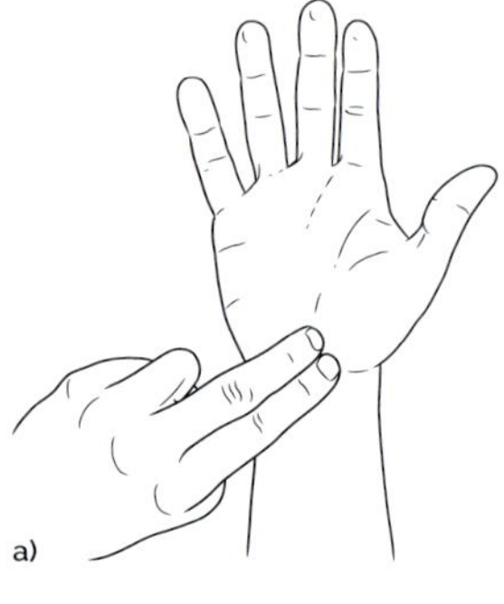

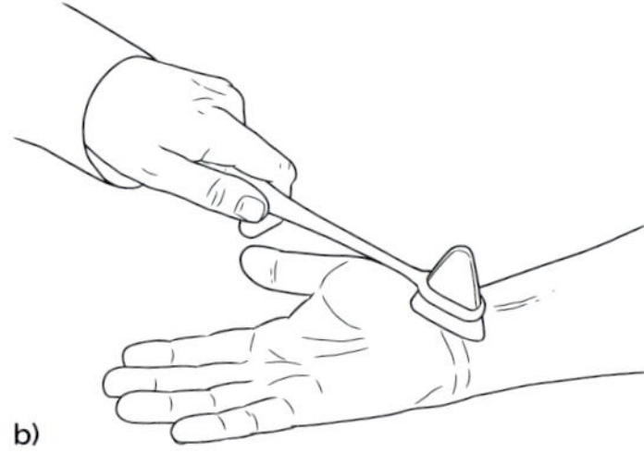

Figure 13.4: Attempting to elicit Tinel's Sign by tapping the carpal tunnel with the fingers (a) or a reflex hammer (b).

Purpose: This tests for carpal tunnel syndrome. Sansone et al. (2006) describe the historic development of this test by Jules Tinel and Paul Hoffmann.

Type of Test: This is a passive neurological test.

Procedure: Begin with your client seated, the wrist supinated and in a neutral position. Tap the midpoint of the carpal tunnel for 60 seconds (figure 13.4a).

Findings: The test is positive if it reproduces the client's symptoms in the sensory distribution pattern of the median nerve: tingling in the thumb, index finger, and middle and lateral half of the ring finger.

Tip: Using a small percussion hammer increases the sensitivity of the test (figure 13.4b).

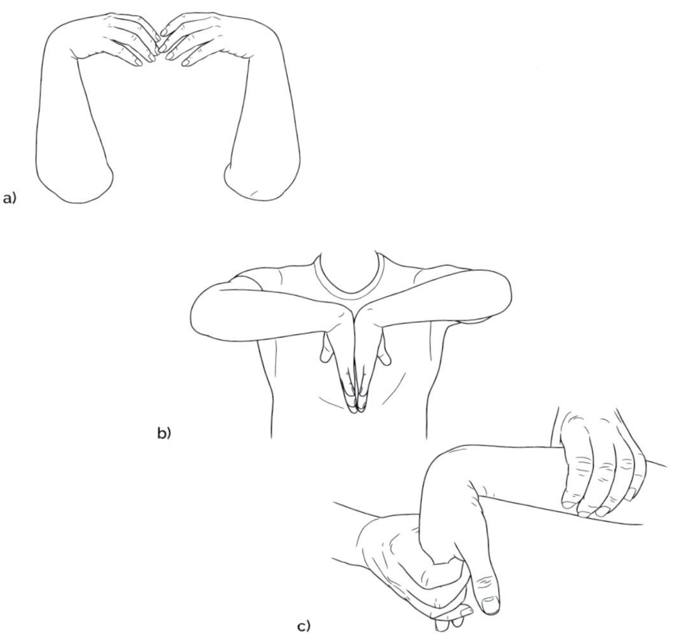

Figure 13.5: Phalen's Test: (a) Phalen's original test position; (b) alternate active position; (c) alternate passive position.

Purpose: This tests for carpal tunnel syndrome. It was described by Phalen, Gardner, and La Londe (1950).

Type of Test: This is a neurological symptom-provocation test that may be performed passively or actively.

Procedure: In the original test described by Phalen, the client was asked to hold their forearms vertically and let their wrists flex (figure 13.5a), holding this position for 30–60 seconds.

The test is commonly performed by asking the client to place the backs of their hands together (figure 13.5b) or by passively flexing the client's wrist (figure 13.5c).

Findings: The test is positive if it reproduces the client's symptoms in the sensory distribution pattern of the median nerve: tingling in the thumb, index finger, and middle and lateral half of the ring finger.

Carpal Compression Test

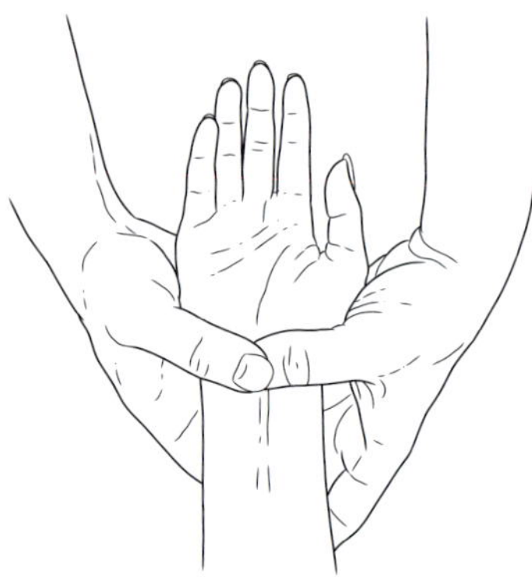

Figure 13.6: Carpal Compression Test.

Purpose: Described by Durkan (1991), this tests for carpal tunnel syndrome (figure 13.6).

Type of Test: This is a passive symptom-provocation neurological test.

Procedure: Begin with your client facing you and their forearm supinated. Apply direct pressure to the median nerve at the wrist.

Findings: The test is positive if it reproduces the client's symptoms in the sensory distribution pattern of the median nerve: tingling in the thumb, index finger, and middle and lateral half of the ring finger.

CHAPTER 14

Thumb Tests

The articulation of the metacarpal bone of the thumb with the trapezium bone of the wrist (figure 14.1a) forms a synovial saddle joint (figure 14.1b). The Grind Test will help you to assess this joint for osteoarthritis. The second test included in this chapter is the Finkelstein Test, which will help you to assess for De Quervain's tenosynovitis, a condition affecting the abductor pollicis longus and extensor pollicis brevis muscles (figure 14.2).

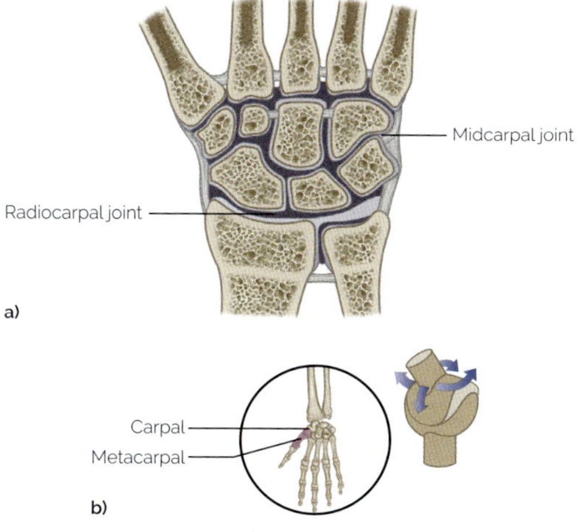

Figure 14.1: The articulation of the metacarpal bone of the thumb with the trapezium bone of the wrist (a) forms a synovial saddle joint (b).

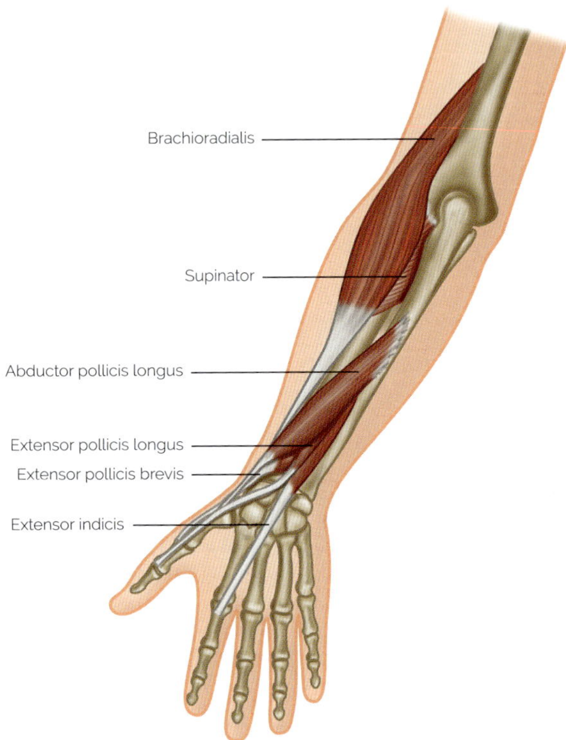

Figure 14.2: Abductor pollicis longus and extensor pollicis brevis muscles of the thumb.

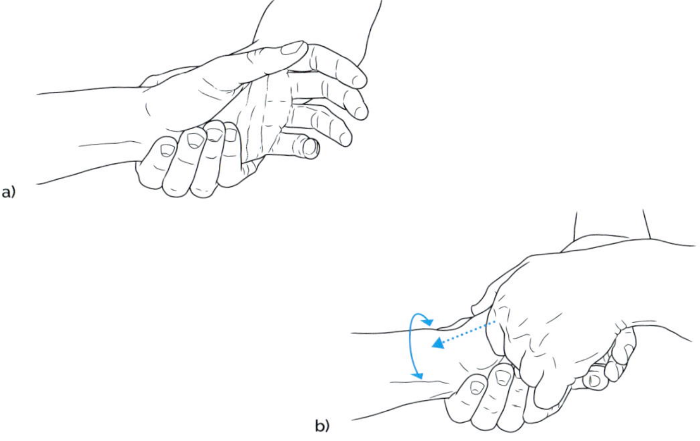

Figure 14.3: Thumb Grind Test: (a) start position; (b) direction of passive movement and pressure.

Purpose: This tests for osteoarthritis at the base of the thumb in the joint between the trapezium and the first metacarpal.

Type of Test: This is a passive pain-provocation test involving compression of the saddle joint of the thumb.

Procedure: The client sits with the ulnar side of their hand resting on a table or treatment plinth, and the wrist in a neutral position. Cup the ulnar side of the client's hand as shown in figure 14.3a. Grasp the metacarpal of the thumb and rotate it back and forth whilst simultaneously applying axial pressure (figure 14.3b).

Findings: The test is positive if there is pain or crepitus at the base of the thumb.

Tip: A useful overview of tests for use in the assessment of thumb osteoarthritis is provided by Normand et al. (2021).

Finkelstein Test

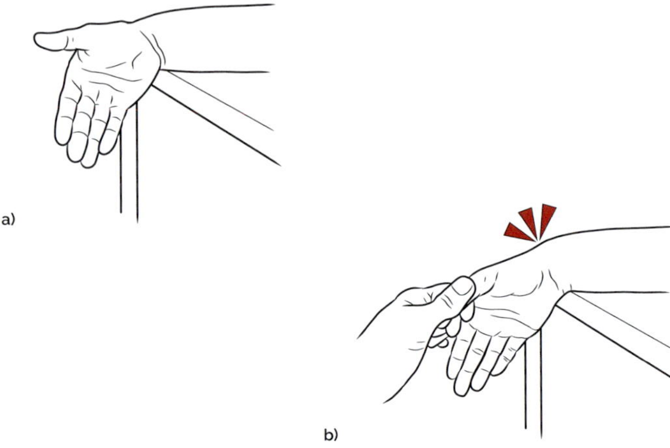

Figure 14.4: Finkelstein Test: (a) beginning with the wrist in ulnar deviation; (b) followed by passive flexion of the thumb.

Purpose: Described by Harry Finkelstein (1930), this tests for De Quervain's tenosynovitis. Wu, Rajpura, and Sandher (2018) note that the instruction manuals and clinicians erroneously describe the Eichhoff test as the Finkelstein test and recommend use of the original Finkelstein test for the diagnosis of De Quervain's disease.

Type of Test: This is a passive pain-provocation test.

Procedure: The client places their wrist on the edge of a table in a position of ulnar deviation (figure 14.4a). You then grasp the client's thumb and passively flex it into the palm (figure 14.4b).

Findings: The test is positive if there is pain over the styloid process.

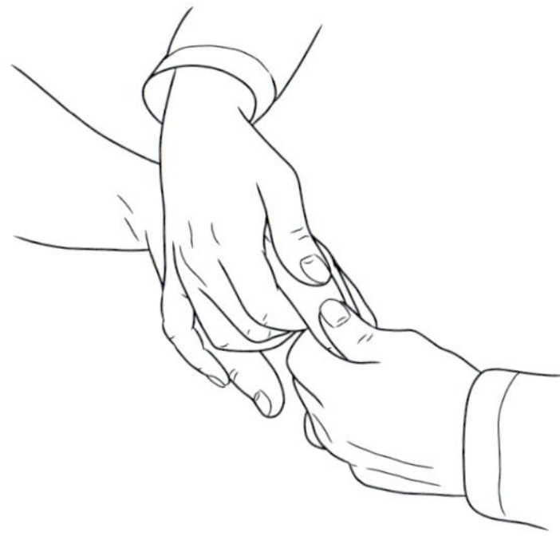

Figure 14.5: Joint Play Movement Test for the Fingers.

Purpose: This tests for movement at the metacarpophalangeal (MCP), proximal interphalangeal (PIP), or distal interphalangeal (DIP) joints of the fingers. Increased movement indicates either hypermobility or injury to the joint, whereas reduced mobility could indicate a condition such as osteoarthritis or soft tissue contracture.

Type of Test: This is a passive joint movement test to discover abnormal stiffness or laxity.

Procedure: Whichever finger joint you aim to test, the procedure is the same. Grasp the finger and isolate the joint in question. You can do this by holding the bones of the joint between your fingers and thumb (figure 14.5).

Findings: The test is determined subjectively by the examiner to identify whether there is increased or decreased movement at the joint being tested.

Tip: This type of test can also be used to assess the MCP joint or the interphalangeal joint of the thumb.

References

Ahsan, Zahab S., Jason E. Hsu, and Albert O. Gee. 2016. "The Snyder classification of superior labrum anterior and posterior (SLAP) lesions." *Clinical Orthopaedics and Related Research* 474 (9): 2075–78.

Allman J. R., and L. Fred. 1967. "Fractures and ligamentous injuries of the clavicle and its articulation." *Journal of Bone and Joint Surgery* 49 (4): 774–84.

Amin, Nirav H., Neil S. Kumar, and Mark S. Schickendantz. 2015. "Medial epicondylitis: Evaluation and management." *Journal of the American Academy of Orthopaedic Surgeons* 23 (6): 348–55.

Antuna, Samuel A., and Shawn W. O'Driscoll. 2001. "Snapping plicae associated with radiocapitellar chondromalacia." *Arthroscopy: The Journal of Arthroscopic and Related Surgery* 17 (5): 491–95.

Barth, Johannes R. H., Stephen S. Burkhart, and Joe F. De Beer. 2006. "The bear-hug test: A new and sensitive test for diagnosing a subscapularis tear." *Arthroscopy: The Journal of Arthroscopic and Related Surgery* 22 (10): 1076–84.

Chalmers, Peter N., Gregory L. Cvetanovich, Noam Kupfer, Markus A. Wimmer, Nikhil N. Verma, Brian J. Cole, Anthony A. Romeo, and Gregory P. Nicholson. 2016. "The champagne toast position isolates the supraspinatus better than the Jobe test: An electromyographic study of shoulder physical examination tests." *Journal of Shoulder and Elbow Surgery* 25 (2): 322–29.

Charles, Edmund R., Vinod Kumar, James Blacknall, Kimberley Edwards, John M. Geoghegan, Paul A. Manning, and W. Angus Wallace. 2017. "A validation of the Nottingham Clavicle Score: A clavicle, acromioclavicular joint and sternoclavicular joint–specific patient-reported outcome measure." *Journal of Shoulder and Elbow Surgery* 26 (10): 1732–39.

Codman, Ernest A. 1934. *The Shoulder: Rupture of the Supraspinatus Tendon and Other Lesions in or about the Subacromial Bursa*. Boston, MA: Thomas Todd.

Dugas, Louis Alexander. 1857. *Report on a New Principle of Diagnosis in Dislocations of the Shoulder-Joint*. Philadelphia, PA: T. K. and P. G. Collins.

Durkan, John A. 1991. "A new diagnostic test for carpal tunnel syndrome." *Journal of Bone and Joint Surgery* 73 (4): 535–38.

Ebinger, Nina, Petra Magosch, Sven Lichtenberg, and Peter Habermeyer. 2008. "A new SLAP test: The supine flexion resistance test." *Arthroscopy: The Journal of Arthroscopic and Related Surgery* 24 (5): 500–505.

Fairbank, S. M., and R. J. Corlett. 2002. "The role of the extensor digitorum communis muscle in lateral epicondylitis." *Journal of Hand Surgery: British and European* 27 (5): 405–9.

Finkelstein, Harry. 1930. "Stenosing tendovaginitis at the radial styloid process." *Journal of Bone and Joint Surgery* 12 (3): 509–40.

Gagey, O. J. 2001. "The hyperabduction test: An assessment of the laxity of the inferior glenohumeral ligament." *Journal of Bone and Joint Surgery: British Volume* 83 (1): 69–74.

Gerber, Christian, and Reinhold Ganz. 1984. "Clinical assessment of instability of the shoulder: With special reference to anterior and posterior drawer tests." *Journal of Bone and Joint Surgery: British Volume* 66 (4): 551–56.

Gerber, Christian, O. Hersche, and A. Farron. 1996. "Isolated rupture of the subscapularis tendon." *Journal of Bone and Joint Surgery: American Volume* 78 (7): 1015–23.

Gerber, Christian, and R. J. Krushell. 1991. "Isolated rupture of the tendon of the subscapularis muscle: Clinical features in 16 cases." *Journal of Bone and Joint Surgery: British Volume* 73 (3): 389–94.

Gerber, Christian, and Richard W. Nyffeler. 2002. "Classification of glenohumeral joint instability." *Clinical Orthopaedics and Related Research (1976–2007)* 400: 65–76.

Gorbaty, Jacob D., Jason E. Hsu, and Albert O. Gee. 2017. "Classifications in brief: Rockwood classification of acromioclavicular joint separations." *Clinical Orthopaedics and Related Research* 475 (1): 283–87.

Hawkins, R. J., and J. C. Kennedy. 1980. "Impingement syndrome in athletes." *American Journal of Sports Medicine* 8 (3): 151–58.

Hertel, R., F. T. Ballmer, S. M. Lambert, and C. H. Gerber. 1996. "Lag signs in the diagnosis of rotator cuff rupture." *Journal of Shoulder and Elbow Surgery* 5 (4): 307–13.

Jobe, Frank W., and Christoper M. Jobe. 1983. "Painful athletic injuries of the shoulder." *Clinical Orthopaedics and Related Research (1976–2007)* 173: 117–24.

Kelly, Bryan T., Warren R. Kadrmas, and Kevin P. Speer. 1996. "The manual muscle examination for rotator cuff strength: An electromyographic investigation." *American Journal of Sports Medicine* 24 (5): 581–88.

Kibler, B. W. 1998. "The role of the scapula in athletic shoulder function." *American Journal of Sports Medicine* 26 (2): 325–37.

Kim, Seung-Ho, Jun-Sic Park, Woong-Kyo Jeong, and Seong-Kee Shin. 2005. "The Kim test: A novel test for posteroinferior labral lesion of the shoulder—a comparison to the jerk test." *American Journal of Sports Medicine* 33 (8): 1188–92.

Kleinman, William B. 2015. "Physical examination of the wrist: Useful provocative maneuvers." *Journal of Hand Surgery* 40 (7): 1486–1500.

Konarski, Wojciech, Tomasz Pobożу, Andrzej Kotela, Martyna Hordowicz, and Kamil Pobożу. 2022. "Ultrasound in the Differential Diagnosis of Medial Epicondylalgia and Medial Elbow Pain—Imaging Findings and Narrative Literature Review." In *Healthcare* 10 (8): 1529.

Ludington, Nelson Amos. 1923. "Rupture of the long head of the biceps flexor cubiti muscle." *Annals of Surgery* 77 (3): 358.

Neer, Charles S. 1983. "Impingement lesions." *Clinical Orthopaedics and Related Research (1976–2007)* 173: 70–77.

Neer, Charles S., and Craig R. Foster. 1980. "*JBJS* Classics: Inferior capsular shift for involuntary inferior and multidirectional instability of the shoulder: A preliminary report." *American Journal of Bone and Joint Surgery* 62A: 897–908.

Normand, Mirka, Tiffany S. Tang, Jean-Michel Brismée, and Stéphane Sobczak. 2021. "Clinical evaluation of thumb base osteoarthritis: A scoping review." *Hand Therapy* 26 (2): 63–78.

O'Brien, Stephen J., Michael J. Pagnani, Stephen Fealy, Scott R. McGlynn, and Joseph B. Wilson. 1998. "The active compression test: A new and effective test for diagnosing labral tears and acromioclavicular joint abnormality." *American Journal of Sports Medicine* 26 (5): 610–13.

O'Driscoll, Shawn W., D. F. Bell, and B. F. Morrey. 1991. "Posterolateral rotatory instability of the elbow." *Journal of Bone and Joint Surgery* 73 (3): 440–46.

O'Driscoll, Shawn W., Lucas B. J. Goncalves, and Patricio Dietz. 2007. "The hook test for distal biceps tendon avulsion." *American Journal of Sports Medicine* 35 (11): 1865–69.

Patte, D., and C. Gerber. 1987. "Pathologie du défilé sous-acromial et coraco-huméral du jeune." In *La pathologie de l'appareil locomoteur liée au sport*, ed. D. Godefroy. Paris: Pfizer.

Pettitt, Robert W., Scott R. Sailor, Gary Lentell, Cary Tanner, and Steven R. Murray. 2008. "Yergason's test: Discrepancies in description and implications for diagnosing biceps subluxation." *Athletic Training Education Journal* 3 (4): 143–47.

Phalen, George S., W. James Gardner, and Albert A. La Londe. 1950. "Neuropathy of the median nerve due to compression beneath the transverse carpal ligament." *Journal of Bone and Joint Surgery* 32 (1): 109–12.

Rabin, Alon, James J. Irrgang, G. Kelley Fitzgerald, and Adam Eubanks. 2006. "The intertester reliability of the scapular assistance test." *Journal of Orthopaedic and Sports Physical Therapy* 36 (9): 653–60.

Roles, N. C., and R. H. Maudsley. 1972. "Radial tunnel syndrome: Resistant tennis elbow as a nerve entrapment." *Journal of Bone and Joint Surgery* 54B: 499–508.

Rowe, Carter R., Donald S. Pierce, and John G. Clark. 1973. "Voluntary dislocation of the shoulder: A preliminary report on a clinical, electromyographic, and psychiatric study of twenty-six patients." *Journal of Bone and Joint Surgery* 55 (3): 445–60.

Sansone, Jason M., Angela M. Gatzke, Florence Aslinia, Loren A. Rolak, and Steven H. Yale. 2006. "Jules Tinel (1879–1952) and Paul Hoffmann (1884–1962)." *Clinical Medicine and Research* 4 (1): 85–89.

Silliman, James F., and Richard J. Hawkins. 1993. "Classification and physical diagnosis of instability of the shoulder." *Clinical Orthopaedics and Related Research (1976–2007)* 291: 7–19.

Siqueira, Mario Gilberto, and Roberto Sergio Martins. 2023. "The Hoffmann-Tinel sign: Historical background and clinical significance." *Arquivos Brasileiros de neurocirurgia: Brazilian Neurosurgery* 43. https://doi.org/10.1055/s-0043-1776273.

Tinel, J. 1971. "The sign of tingling in lesions of the peripheral nerves." *Archives of Neurology* 24 (6): 574–75.

Tossy, Jerome D., Newton C. Mead, and Harley M. Sigmond. 1963. "11 acromioclavicular separations: Useful and practical classification for treatment." *Clinical Orthopaedics and Related Research (1976–2007)* 28: 111–19.

Tuhi, Rebecca. 2023. "Diagnostic accuracy in the clinical examination for identifying a triangular fibrocartilage complex injury." MPhil thesis, Auckland University of Technology.

Vezeridis, Peter S., Hiroshi Yoshioka, Roger Han, and Philip Blazar. 2010. "Ulnar-sided wrist pain. Part I: Anatomy and physical examination." *Skeletal Radiology* 39: 733–45.

Walton, Judie, Sanjeev Mahajan, Anastasios Paxinos, Jeanette Marshall, Carl Bryant, Ron Shnier, Richard Quinn, and George AC Murrell. 2004. "Diagnostic values of tests for acromioclavicular joint pain." *Journal of Bone and Joint Surgery* 86 (4): 807–12.

Watson, H. Kirk, D.T.I.V. Ashmead, and M. Vincent Makhlouf. 1988. "Examination of the scaphoid." *Journal of Hand Surgery* 13 (5): 657–60.

Wu, Feiran, Asim Rajpura, and Dilraj Sandher. 2018. "Finkelstein's test is superior to Eichhoff's test in the investigation of de Quervain's disease." *Journal of Hand and Microsurgery* 10 (2): 116–18.

Yergason, R. M. 1931. "Supination sign." *Journal of Bone and Joint Surgery* 13: 160.

Zaslav, Kenneth R. 2001. "Internal rotation resistance strength test: A new diagnostic test to differentiate intra-articular pathology from outlet (Neer) impingement syndrome in the shoulder." *Journal of Shoulder and Elbow Surgery* 10 (1): 23–27.

Appendix

Test	Rationale for Use	Page Reference
Shoulder		
AC Joint Mobility Test	Laxity in the AC joint	12
AC Shear Test	AC joint pathology	13
Active Compression Test	See *O'Brien's Test*	
Anterior Drawer Test	Instability of the glenohumeral joint, specifically laxity in the anterior shoulder capsule	68
Anterior Instability Apprehension Test	Instability of the glenohumeral joint	67
Apley's Scratch Test	Range of movement in the shoulder	21
Bear Hug Test	Lesions of subscapularis	40
Belly Press Test	Integrity of subscapularis	37
Belly Off Sign	Lesions of subscapularis	39
Biceps Load Test 1	SLAP lesions in people with anterior shoulder instability	54
Biceps Load Test 2	SLAP lesions	55
Champagne Toast Test	Supraspinatus tendon pathology	28
Clunk Test	SLAP lesions	51
Codman's Test	See *Drop Arm Test*	
Compression Rotation Test	See *Crank Test*	
Crank Test	SLAP Lesions	50
Cross Body Adduction Stress Test	See *Scarf Test*	
Drop Arm Test	Weakness and lesion of supraspinatus	32
Dugas Test	Anterior dislocation of the glenohumeral joint	65
Empty Can Test	See *Jobe's Test*	
External Rotation Lag Sign	Rupture of infraspinatus and supraspinatus tendons	42

Test	Rationale for Use	Page Reference
Fulcrum Test	Glenohumeral anterior instability	69
Full Can Test	Strength of supraspinatus Integrity of the supraspinatus tendon	30
Gagey Hyperabduction Test	Integrity of the inferior glenohumeral ligament	64
Gerber's Lift Off Test	Damage and/or weakness of	35
Habermeyer's Supine Flexion Resistance Test	SLAP lesions	49
Hawkins-Kennedy Test	Subacromial impingement pain	27
Hertel's Drop Sign	Lesions of infraspinatus	43
Internal Rotation Lag Sign	Full-thickness tears of subscapularis	36
Internal Rotation Resistance Strength Test	To differentiate between intra-articular pathology and impingement of the supraspinatus tendon	46
Jerk Test	Posterior instability of the glenohumeral joint	72
Jobe's Test	Posterior-inferior labral tears Damage and/or weakness to the supraspinatus muscle or tendon	29
Kim's Test	Posterior-inferior lesion of the glenohumeral labrum	52
Lateral Scapular Slide Test	Stability of the scapula during movement of the glenohumeral joint	22
Load and Shift Test	Laxity of the humeral head in the glenohumeral fossa	66
Ludington's Test	Proximal biceps brachii tendinopathy or rupture	58
Napoleon Sign	Integrity of subscapularis	38
Neer's Impingement Sign	Subacromial impingement lesions of the supraspinatus tendon Pathology affecting the subacromial bursa, long head of biceps brachii, and other rotator cuff structures	33

Test	Rationale for Use	Page Reference
Neer's Test	Inferior instability of the glenohumeral joint	62
O'Brien's Test	Lesions of the AC joint and glenohumeral joint	16
Painful Arc Test	AC joint and supraspinatus pathology	18, 26
Patte's Test	Integrity of teres minor	45
Paxino's Test	AC joint pathology	14
Posterior Apprehension Test	Posterior instability of the glenohumeral joint	70
Posterior Drawer Test	Subluxation of the glenohumeral joint	71
Resisted AC Joint Extension Test	AC joint pathology	17
Rowe's Test	Inferior subluxation of the shoulder	63
Scapular Assistance Test	Whether impingement at the shoulder may be due to lack of active acromial elevation	24
Scarf Test	Integrity of the AC joint	15
Speed's Test	Tenosynovitis of the long tendon of biceps brachii	57
Sulcus Sign	See *Neer's Test*	
Walch's Hornblower Sign	Pathology affecting teres minor and infraspinatus	44
Yergason's Test	Biceps brachii tendon pathology SLAP lesions	56
Yocum's Test	Subacromial impingement	31
Elbow		
Chair Push-Up Test	Posterolateral rotatory instability of the elbow Integrity of the lateral collateral ligament of the elbow	90
Cozen's Test	Lateral epicondylalgia	80
Elbow Hook Test	Rupture of the distal tendon of biceps brachii	101

Test	Rationale for Use	Page Reference
Elbow Plica Entrapment (Extension-Supination) Test	Entrapment of the posterior plica of the elbow	100
Elbow Plica Entrapment (Flexion-Pronation) Test	Entrapment of the lateral plica of the elbow	99
Golfer's Elbow Provocation Test	Medial epicondylalgia	78
Golfer's Elbow Test	Medial epicondylalgia	79
Maudsley's Test	Lateral epicondylalgia	82
Mill's Test	Lateral epicondylalgia Radial nerve stress test	81
Moving Valgus Stress Test	Instability of the medial collateral ligament of the elbow	88
Polk's Test	Differentiation between lateral and medial epicondylalgia	83
Posterolateral Rotatory-Instability Test	Posterolateral rotatory instability of the elbow Integrity of the lateral collateral ligament of the elbow	89
Pressure Provocation Test	Cubital tunnel syndrome	95
Supinator Compression Test	Entrapment of the deep branch of the radial nerve at the arcade of Frohse	97
Tinel's Test or Hoffman-Tinel Sign	Cubital tunnel syndrome	96
Ulnar Nerve Flexion Test	Cubital tunnel syndrome	94
Valgus Stress Test	Medial collateral ligament of the elbow	86
Varus Stress Test	Lateral collateral ligament of the elbow	87
Wrist		
Carpal Compression Test	Carpal tunnel syndrome	122
Dorsal Capitate Displacement Apprehension Test	Stability of the capitate bone	116

Test	Rationale for Use	Page Reference
Lunotriquetral Shear Test	Integrity of the lunotriquetral ligament	112
Lunotriquetral Shear Test (Kleinman)	Instability of the lunotriquetral joint	113
Lunotriquetral Shear Test (Linscheid)	Integrity of the lunotriquetral ligament	115
Lunotriquetral Shear Test (Raegan)	Integrity of the lunotriquetral ligament	114
Phalen's Test	Carpal Tunnel Syndrome	121
Piano Key Test	Integrity of the distal radio-ulnar joint	109
Radial Collateral Ligament Stress Test	Integrity of the radial collateral ligament	107
Scaphoid Shift Test	See *Watson Test*	
Supination Lift Test	Integrity of the TFCC	117
Tinel's Sign Test	Carpal tunnel syndrome	120
Ulnar Collateral Ligament Stress Test	Integrity of the ulnar collateral ligament	108
Watson Test	Integrity of the scapholunate ligament	110
Fingers/Thumb		
Axial Compression Test	See *Thumb Grind Test*	
Finkelstein Test	De Quervain's tenosynovitis subscapularis	126
Joint Play Movement Test for Fingers	Movement at the MCP, PIP or DIP joints of the fingers	127
Thumb Grind Test	Osteoarthritis between the trapezium and first metacarpal	125